Deep vein thrombosis and pulmonary embolism

A guide for practitioners

Deep vein thrombosis and pulmonary embolism

A guide for practitioners

Dr Andrew Blann

Deep vein thrombosis and pulmonary embolism: a guide for practitioners 2nd edition

Andrew Blann

ISBN: 9781905539-33-8

First published 2009; this revised edition published 2015

British Library Cataloguing in Publication Data

A catalogue record for this book is available from the British Library

Notice

Clinical practice and medical knowledge constantly evolve. Standard safety precautions must be followed, but, as knowledge is broadened by research, changes in practice, treatment and drug therapy may become necessary or appropriate. Readers must check the most current product information provided by the manufacturer of each drug to be administered and verify the dosages and correct administration, as well as contraindications. It is the responsibility of the practitioner, utilising the experience and knowledge of the patient, to determine dosages and the best treatment for each individual patient. Any brands mentioned in this book are as examples only and are not endorsed by the publisher. Neither the publisher nor the authors assume any liability for any injury and/or damage to persons or property arising from this publication.

Disclaimer

M&K Publishing cannot accept responsibility for the contents of any linked website or online resource. The existence of a link does not imply any endorsement or recommendation of the organisation or the information or views which may be expressed in any linked website or online resource. We cannot guarantee that these links will operate consistently and we have no control over the availability of linked pages.

To contact M&K Publishing write to:
M&K Update Ltd · The Old Bakery · St. John's Street
Keswick · Cumbria CA12 5AS
Tel: 01768 773030 · Fax: 01768 781099
publishing@mkupdate.co.uk
www.mkupdate.co.uk

Designed and typeset by Mary Blood
Printed in Scotland by Bell & Bain, Glasgow

Contents

Figures

Tables

About the author

Dr Andrew Blann PhD FRCPath FCRP (Ed)
is Consultant Clinical Scientist and Honorary Senior Lecturer in Medicine
at University Department of Medicine, City Hospital, Birmingham, UK

Introduction

Venous thromboembolism

Many common problems in clinical medicine and general practice relate to arterial and venous thrombosis. Thrombosis in veins (i.e. **venous thromboembolism: VTE***) is a permanent problem in various cancers and following surgery, especially orthopaedic. Other risk factors include diabetes, smoking and obesity. It has been estimated that deaths due to VTE in the European Community exceed those due to AIDS, breast cancer, prostate cancer and road traffic accidents *combined*.

Pathology

A clot (**thrombus**) may consist simply of blood **platelets** stuck together with the glue-like **fibrin**, although red blood cells and white blood cells may also get caught up in the clot. A thrombus may form in the blood, or may develop from, and stick to, the inside of the blood vessel, from which anchored point it may grow. However, fragments (**emboli**) of this anchored clot may break off and fly away into the blood to cause problems elsewhere.

Recognition

The problem areas are clots in veins of the leg (**deep vein thrombosis: DVT**) and clots in the lungs (**pulmonary embolus: PE**) – clearly, each have their own different sets of signs and symptoms. These conditions are very well recognised and there are several aids to diagnosis, such as probability scores and laboratory tests. Together, DVTs and PEs comprise 95% of all VTEs; the remaining clots are most commonly found in the veins of the arms and shoulders.

Prevention and treatment

Ideally, prevention of VTE is by the avoidance (or minimisation) of risk factors such as poor diet and lack of exercise, but if this is impossible (e.g. surgery, cancer), there are drug and non-drug treatments which are also used once a clot is present.

Anti-thrombotic agents have been developed and the many classes of agents that are available are an attempt to find solutions to the wide range of thrombus-related disorders needing treatment. Until recently, the agents most commonly used in **prophylaxis** and treatment of VTE are **heparin**, **low molecular weight heparin** (**LMWH**) and a **vitamin K antagonist** (almost always **warfarin**). However, a new class of drugs, the non-vitamin K antagonist oral anticoagulants (**NOACs**), also known as direct-acting oral coagulants (**DOACs**), are set to take over from these traditional drugs in several conditions. Another group of drugs, such as streptokinase, may be used in an attempt to destroy or lyse the clot once it has been formed (i.e. thrombolysis). In the UK, the National Institute for Health and Care Excellence (NICE) is the dominant regulatory body, issuing advice, appraisals and guidance on the diagnosis and management of VTE.

*Key words, when first mentioned, are formatted in bold and are explained in the Glossary (page 88).

Chapter 1

What are deep vein thrombosis and pulmonary embolism and why are they important?

Clots often get a bad press, but their place in physiology is essential in minimising blood loss (**haemorrhage**). The process of healthy clot formation, **coagulation**, is generally very tightly regulated, but when this control goes wrong it can lead to build-up of clot that can then lead to clinically important thrombosis, which may even be fatal, especially if in the lung.

How coagulation works

A clot (thrombus) is formed from the platelet and fibrin. Platelets are tiny bodies produced (like red and white blood cells) in the bone marrow. The glue-like fibrin is formed from fibrinogen, produced by the liver. Fibrinogen is converted into fibrin by the crucial clotting enzyme thrombin, a molecule so active that it cannot exist by itself in the plasma, but circulates in blood in an inactive form as prothrombin, which is also produced by the liver. Prothrombin is converted to thrombin by a collection of other coagulation factors (**Factor VII**, **Factor X**, calcium) and molecules that together are known as the prothrombinase complex.

Many of us will be aware of the most well-known bleeding disease, **haemophilia**. This is caused by the lack of a particular coagulation protein, **Factor VIII**. The coagulation pathway itself is generally a well-regulated cascade of some 20 such coagulation factors, all acting in strict order. Fortunately, it is not important to know the full workings of this pathway in order to be a fully competent Thrombosis Practitioner. However, for completeness, Figure 1.1 shows how these many different molecules act together to generate a fibrin clot.

The coagulation pathway cannot run unchecked, otherwise we would all clot to death. A series of regulators keep the coagulation pathway in check. The principal inhibitors are **antithrombin**, **protein S** and **protein C**, all produced by the liver. They become activated a few crucial seconds after the coagulation pathway itself becomes activated, and eventually catch it up and then close it down.

Once a clot has been formed, and it has done its job, it must be removed by a process called

fibrinolysis. This is done by the blood enzyme **plasmin**, which digests the fibrin strands. These bits of chopped-up clots in the plasma can be detected in the laboratory, and of these fragments, D-dimers are the most useful. Thus increased **D-dimers** are evidence of fibrinolysis, and so of the presence of a clot being resolved. It follows that an increased D-dimer result is indicative of thrombotic disease.

Coagulation is a dynamic process. The view that clotting stops and starts in a very defined way, with exact on/off signals, is now becoming obsolete. The current view suggests that we are all clotting ourselves all the time, all over the body. Fortunately, we are also dissolving these clots just as fast (by fibrinolysis) so that they do not (generally) become a problem. However, if the clot-making pathway is quicker or more effective than the clot-inhibiting and clot-breaking pathways, then thrombosis can occur.

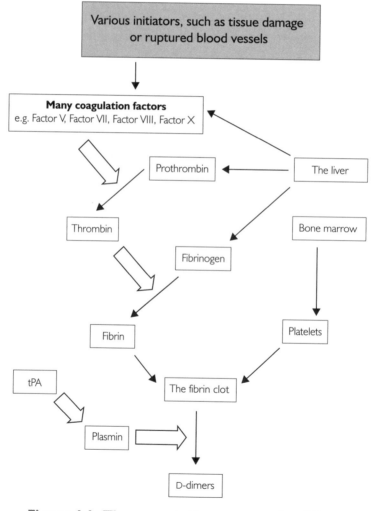

Figure 1.1 The coagulation system simplified

Legend to Figure 1.1

Several factors start the coagulation 'cascade', such as crush injuries, severe bacterial infections or severed blood vessels that expose collagen. Among the first coagulation factors to be activated are Factor V and Factor VII. A major inhibitor of Factor V is Protein C.

Later, Factor X becomes activated and so is referred to as **Factor Xa**. The activity of this molecule is inhibited by LMWH and some members of the NOAC class of drugs, and Factor Xa is a major contributor to the complex of Factors and other molecules that form a so-called 'prothombinase' complex, the function of which is to convert prothrombin into thrombin.

Once formed, thrombin acts on fibrinogen to turn it into fibrin. However, the activity of thrombin is regulated by another inhibitor, anti-thrombin. Heparin works by promoting the activity of anti-thrombin. Fibrin forms a mesh that, with platelets and other blood cells, generates a thrombus (clot) to reduce blood flow.

Fibrinolysis is the dissolution of a clot. A thrombus is digested by the enzyme plasmin, which needs to be activated by **tissue plasminogen activator (tPA)**. The products of the digestion of a fibrin clot are D-dimers.

Small arrows indicate direct pathways in clot formation. Large open arrows indicate the action of enzyme activators of coagulation (the 'prothombinase' complex, thrombin) and of fibrinolysis (tPA, plasmin).

Haemostasis is therefore the overall balance between coagulation (thrombus formation) and fibrinolysis (thrombus removal):

● When the balance falls in favour of coagulation, the result is thrombosis.
● When the balance falls in favour of fibrinolysis, the result is haemorrhage.

Venous thrombosis: What is it?

Good haemostasis is not a problem. However, disease follows irregularities in this process of clot formation and removal – haemorrhage when clots are not formed, and thrombosis when too many or too large a clot is formed too rapidly. Thrombosis can occur in the arteries or in the veins, the latter being a **venous thromboembolism (VTE)**, which is also sometimes known as veno-thromboembolism or a veno-thromboembolic event. Thrombosis is more likely to happen in conditions of increased numbers of platelets and high levels of fibrinogen, the inappropriate activation of the entire system, and/or the lack or ineffectiveness of inhibitors. Both high numbers of platelets and raised fibrinogen are present in smoking, hypertension, diabetes and dyslipidaemia. These are, of course, the risk factors for arterial thrombosis and atherosclerosis. Obesity is an important modifiable risk factor for VTE.

Clots in the veins (i.e. VTE) are somewhat different from those in arteries; there are more risk factors but the clots are generally in only two places: the legs and groin (where a deep vein thrombosis (DVT) can develop) and the vessels of the lung (where a pulmonary embolus (PE) may arise). Rarely, the subclavian and mesenteric vessels, and the abdominal vena cava are burdened. DVT generally includes the large saphenous and femoral veins although some classify calf vein thrombosis separately.

Why are DVT and PE important?

Not only do DVT and PE lead to considerable morbidity, clots also kill!

- A DVT leads to a swollen, painful leg such that walking can be difficult, perhaps impossible. DVTs by themselves are rarely fatal but can produce considerable long-term morbidity. There is also powerful evidence that DVT seeds PE. Approximately three-quarters of all VTEs are DVT.

- Blockage of a crucial lung vessel (be it an artery or a vein) by a PE will lead to breathlessness and pain, can lead in the long term to congestive lung disease and heart disease, and can indeed be fatal. PEs make up about a quarter of all VTEs.

But how big a problem is VTE and who is likely to suffer an event? In a UK study from 1989, about 10% of hospital deaths (1% of admissions) were attributable to PE. However, lower limb DVT has been documented in 50% of major orthopaedic operations performed without anti-thrombotic prophylaxis, in 25% of patients with acute myocardial infarction and in more than 50% of acute ischaemic stroke cases.

VTE is far from a benign condition. Ten years after thrombosis:

- Over half the patients will have suffered post-thrombotic syndrome. This is a late consequence of DVT. Clinical signs are chronic leg pain, cramps, varicose veins, redness, swelling, eczema, dermatitis etc., and often follows valve destruction. Leg ulcers (present in 0.2% of the general population) are observed in 2–10% of patients ~10 years after their first symptomatic DVT.

- Over a quarter will have suffered a recurrent VTE.
  Over a quarter will be dead, mostly from cancer, congestive lung disease, myocardial infarction or stroke.

Consolidation (see pages 82–85 for answers)

1.1 What are the two major constituents of a clot?

1.2 What are the two major coagulation factors in the blood?

1.3 What is the name for the process of clot destruction?

1.4 What product of clot destruction can be measured in the plasma?

Chapter 2

Who is at risk of these conditions and why?

The many causes of DVT and PE can be divided into two groups: those which are hereditary and those which are acquired. A clear clinical risk factor for thrombosis can often be identified in over 80% of patients, but there is often more than one factor at play in a given patient. The most common include the following:

The elderly

Epidemiology studies suggest a rate of 100 per 100,000 people (0.1%) per year in the general population that translates to some 55,000 cases annually. This rate is strongly influenced by age: <5 per 100,000 teenagers, 30 per 100,000 in 25–35-year-olds, to 500 per 100,000 80-year-olds. This may be due to immobility and/or coagulopathy.

Major general surgery

The risk of VTE after major general surgery has been extensively documented – it generally includes abdominal and thoracic surgery requiring general anaesthesia of over 30 minutes. Examples of this include coronary artery bypass grafting, surgery for gynaecological malignancies, and major urological surgery.

Major orthopaedic surgery and other bone trauma

Lower extremity orthopaedic operations such as total hip and knee replacement carry a particular high risk and, without prophylaxis, about 50% develop VTE. Arthroscopy is of particularly low risk, so that prophylaxis is optional, dependent on other risk factors. VTE is common in fracture of the pelvis, hip or long bones. Indeed, in one of the first trials of an anticoagulant, the incidence of death from PE after hip fracture fell from 10% to zero!

Cancer

VTE is a frequent complication in patients with cancer and represents a common clinical problem, often preceding diagnosis of cancer by months or years. In the past, patients with cancer were nearly twice as likely to die of PE as those with benign disease and about 60% of these deaths occur prematurely. In one community study the one-year survival of those with cancer and a VTE was 12%, compared to 36% in those with cancer but no VTE.

Patients with cancer represent maybe 15–20% of all new cases of VTE occurring in the community. Conversely, perhaps 10% of people with idiopathic VTEs are ultimately diagnosed with cancer within the year, and VTEs appear to be particularly predominant in lymphoma, carcinoma of the pancreas, ovary, breast, lung, brain, pelvis, rectum and gastrointestinal tract.

Therapeutic interventions in patients with cancer, especially surgery and **chemotherapy** (such as **cytotoxic drugs**) further increase the risk for thrombosis. Indeed, patients may need anticoagulation prophylaxis during cycles of cytotoxic chemotherapy. Formal guidelines are becoming available (see 'Selected references').

Pregnancy, the puerperium and synthetic hormones

The incidence of VTE in healthy young women not taking an oral contraceptive pill (OCP) is about 0.5 to 1 per 10,000 per year. Use of a low-dose OCP gives a 3- to 5-fold risk increase (e.g. to 2.5 per 10,000). Almost all these VTEs are DVT, and so are rarely fatal.

Pregnancy increases VTE risk considerably (i.e. to 5 in 10,000). PE is a leading cause of death after childbirth, with 10 events per 10,000 births, although only one of these is likely to be fatal. The risk of DVT following childbirth rises to 20 times that of age-matched non-pregnant women, and is raised even higher by smoking and a history of previous VTE.

The risk of VTE in hormone replacement therapy (HRT) is 2- to 4-fold compared to age-matched controls. Women with a history of VTE who are using HRT are at greater risk of recurrence than those not on HRT. Interestingly, men on **oestrogens** for prostate cancer are also at an increased risk of VTE. A note on practical aspects of risk. Suppose the risk of a DVT on one type of OCP is 15 per 100,000. This translates to one woman getting a VTE from 6,667 women on that pill. Whether or not this risk is acceptable depends on the woman!

The frequencies of these and other risk factors are presented in Table 2.1.

Thrombophilia

A separate condition has been described for the appearance of a VTE in 20% of people who lack a clear risk factor (i.e. those above). This condition is called **thrombophilia** (literally, 'clot loving'), and is typically suspected in a slim young woman not on the oral contraceptive pill whose clot appears 'out of the blue', especially if she has a family history of VTE. The most common reasons for thrombophilia are genetic, and in the vast majority of cases are inherited (Table 2.2), although some can be acquired.

Factor V Leiden is the most common genetic cause of unexplained VTE, and has a remarkable evolutionary history. In its **heterozygous** state it is prevalent in about 5% of the population of north-west Europe, North America, Australia, (white) South Africa and New Zealand, with lesser incidence in India and Pakistan and in some black populations in Africa. It leads to a seven-fold increase in the risk of VTE and is present in about 20% of unselected, consecutive patients with DVT.

Table 2.1 Risk factors in 1231 patients with VTE

Risk factor	%	Risk factor	%
Age >40 years	88.5	Obesity	37.8
History of VTE	26.0	Cancer	22.3
Bed rest >5 days	12.0	Major surgery	11.2
Congestive heart failure	8.2	Varicose veins	5.8
Hip or leg fracture	3.7	Oestrogen use	2.0
Stroke	1.8	Multiple trauma	1.1
Childbirth	1.1	Myocardial infarction	0.7

One or more risks present in 96% of subjects
Two or more risks in 76%, and three or more risks in 39%

(Modified from Anderson & Wheeler 1992)

Table 2.2
Prevalence of inherited risk factors for VTE in Caucasians

Risk factor	Prevalence in the general population (%)	Prevalence in patients with VTE
Factor V Leiden	5	High
Prothrombin gene mutation	2	Moderate
Protein S deficiency	0.7	Low
Protein C deficiency	0.2–0.4	Low
Anti-thrombin deficiency	0.02	Low

Other contributors to thrombophilia include high coagulation Factor VIII, and **anti-phospholipid antibodies**. Many such conditions are hereditary, so family history may be relevant. Therefore thrombosis can occur if there is a problem not simply with excess generation of a clot, but also with the lack of inhibitors (Proteins C and S, anti-thrombin) that would normally limit the development of such a thrombosis. These problems are compounded in the rare and unfortunate person who lacks more than one inhibitor. Thus those with dual Factor V Leiden and anti-thrombin deficiency are at very high risk of thrombosis.

However, not all VTE risk factors are equal; some are more dangerous than others (Table 2.3). Furthermore, the risk of VTE is often additive in the presence of several risk factors. One research paper reported an increased risk of VTE of 2.4 times in the obese (BMI >30). A combination of obesity and Factor V Leiden brings a risk of 7.9 times. However, the risk of VTE in an obese woman using oral contraceptives is 23.8 times that of a normal BMI woman not on the pill.

Table 2.3 Risk factor stratification

Strong risk factors (increased risk >10)
Hip, pelvis or leg fracture, hip or knee replacement, major general surgery (e.g. coronary artery bypass graft), major trauma, spinal cord injury.
Moderate risk factors (increased risk 2–9)
Arthroscopic knee surgery, central venous lines, malignancy (alone, 4 times, but with chemotherapy this rises to 6 times), congestive heart or respiratory failure, HRT, use of oral contraceptives, paralytic stroke, post-partum pregnancy, previous VTE, thrombophilia.
Weak risk factors (increased risk <2)
Bed rest >3 days, immobility due to sitting (e.g. prolonged car or air travel, wheelchair), increasing age, laparoscopic surgery (e.g. cholecystectomy), obesity, ante-partum pregnancy, varicose veins.

Consolidation (see pages 82–85 for answers)

2.1 Describe some surgical procedures that carry a strong risk of DVT or PE.

2.2 Which risk factors are generally relevant only to women?

2.3 Why do some risk factors seem to promote thrombosis?

2.4 What genetic condition is the most common cause of thrombophilia?

Chapter 3

Recognising and confirming VTE

Almost all VTEs are either DVT or PE (and sometimes both). Diagnosis of VTE based on clinical observation alone is of poor accuracy; in DVT it is correct in only 25–33% of cases so that the practitioner must be aware of differential diagnoses. However, other aids are available: compression ultrasonography and contrast venography for DVT, ventilation perfusion scan for PE, and the blood test D-dimers for both types of VTE. These improve the likelihood of making a correct diagnosis. Sections of NICE CG144 are relevant.

Recognising DVT

Clinical signs

The problem is with the presenting patient, who may give a difficult and/or vague history and symptoms. What exactly is the problem? Always consider alternative diagnoses: it may not be a DVT. Possible non-DVT causes of pain or swelling of the leg include:

- superficial phlebitis, post-thrombotic syndrome, chronic venous insufficiency and venous obstruction
- cellulitis, Baker's cyst, torn gastrocnemius muscle, fracture, haematoma
- acute arterial ischaemia, lymphoedema and hypoproteinaemia (for example, in cirrhosis).

Since well under half of patients presenting with a suspected DVT actually have the condition, a reliable algorithm for differential diagnosis is needed.

DVT commonly presents with pain, erythema, tenderness and swelling of the affected limb. Findings on examination include a palpable cord (reflecting a thrombosed vein), warmth, oedema or superficial venous dilatation. Non-deep veins include those of the calf. Objective diagnosis of DVT (as with PE) is important for best management, and although clinical diagnosis is imprecise, models based on clinical features are fairly practical and reliable in predicting the likelihood of an event.

Imaging

Compression ultrasonography remains the non-invasive tool of choice for the investigation and diagnosis of clinically suspected DVT. Although such imaging is highly sensitive for detecting proximal (groin (iliac) and upper leg (saphenous)) DVT, it is less accurate in the case of isolated DVT of the calf. The ideal method, invasive contrast angiography, is used when a definitive answer is required. Newer imaging techniques being developed (for example, magnetic resonance venography, computed tomography) could detect pelvic vein thromboses, although further testing is necessary to establish their role in the diagnosis of DVT.

D-dimers

This blood test adds to the diagnostic accuracy of the non-invasive tests as levels are high in nearly all patients with a VTE. However, several common conditions also lead to raised D-dimers, such as cancer, atherosclerosis, smoking, obesity and diabetes.

Thus, a low or normal D-dimer with a low pre-test probability makes a diagnosis of DVT (or, indeed, of PE) unlikely and therefore excludes this possible diagnosis.

The Wells score for DVT

For assessment of pre-test probability of a suspected DVT:

● Score 1 point each for the following: tenderness along the entire deep vein system, swelling of the entire leg, greater than 3cm difference in calf circumference, pitting oedema, collateral superficial veins, risk factors present (active cancer, prolonged immobility or paralysis, recent surgery or major medical illness).

● Subtract 2 points for an alternative diagnosis likely (e.g. as above: ruptured Baker's cyst in rheumatoid arthritis, superficial thrombophlebitis or infective cellulitis).

● Result: Greater than 3: High probability
           1–2:   Moderate probability
           0 or less: Low probability

Figure 3.1 shows a practical approach to the diagnosis of DVT using the pre-test probability model, ultrasound, D-dimers and a clinical approach to diagnosis.

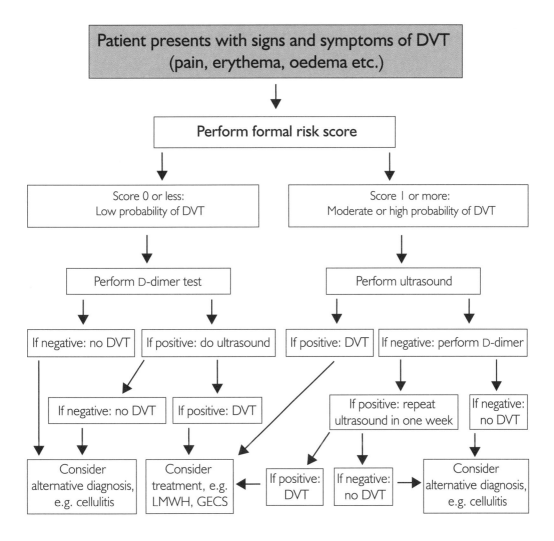

Figure 3.1

A clinical approach to the diagnosis of possible DVT

Recognising PE

Those presenting with sudden onset of breathlessness with haemoptysis, pleuritic chest pain, or collapse with shock, in the absence of other causes, should be investigated urgently, as PE has a high risk of mortality and morbidity. Most patients have no leg symptoms at diagnosis, with less than a third having signs or symptoms of a DVT. Conversely, many patients with symptomatic DVT may have asymptomatic PE. Given the common pathophysiology, this is not surprising. Indeed, it has been suggested that 90% of cases arise from asymptomatic DVT.

A similar clinical model to that for DVT has been developed for PE. This model considers the most common symptoms of:

- dyspnoea, present in 73%
- pleuritic pain, present in 66%
- cough, present in 37%

and the most common signs of:

- tachypnoea, present in 70%
- crepitations, present in 51%
- tachycardia, present in 30%.

In severe PE, circulatory collapse, atrial fibrillation and cardiac arrest may occur. Probably the ultimate diagnostic tool for PE is the ventilation-perfusion (VQ) scan. However, this may not always be available. Accordingly, as for DVT, a scoring system for PE has been devised.

The Wells score for PE

- Score three points for each of the clinical features of DVT and no alternative explanation for acute breathlessness or pleuritic chest pain.
- Score 1.5 points for each of recent prolonged immobility or surgery in the previous 4 weeks, previous history of DVT or PE, and resting heart rate >100 bpm.
- Score 1 point for each of active cancer and haemoptysis.
- Result: Greater than 6.0: High probability
  2.0–6.0: Moderate probability
  1.5 or less: Low probability

Measurement of D-dimer levels, as used for DVT, is helpful, especially when combined with other markers. Figure 3.2 shows a practical approach to the diagnosis of PE using a number of factors: the pretest probability model, imaging, the laboratory, and a clinical approach to diagnosis, although other pretest models exist.

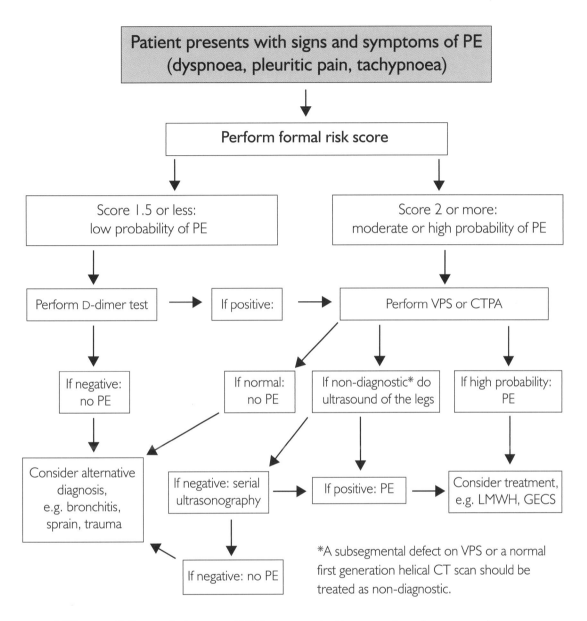

VPS = ventilation perfusion scan, CTPA = computed tomography pulmonary angiogram.

Figure 3.2
A clinical approach to the diagnosis of possible PE

Consolidation (see pages 82–85 for answers)

3.1 What are the most common clinical signs and symptoms of DVT?

3.2 What other aids are there to help diagnosis?

3.3 What are the most common signs and symptoms of PE?

3.4 What other aids are there to help diagnosis?

Case Study 1

A 65-year-old woman with type II diabetes and a body mass index of 32.9 presents to A&E with a 24-hour history of pain, tenderness and swelling in the left leg. The circumference of the left calf is 2cm greater than the right. Chest sounds are normal and she has no pain or cough. Blood pressures are 123/76mmHg, pulse rate 77bpm. A venous blood sample is obtained and sent to the laboratory, with the result of no evidence of systemic inflammation. However, the level of D-dimers is raised at 750 units/mL (normal range <500 units/mL).

What action would you take?

Chapter 4

What have we got to treat these conditions?

Clearly, step one in reducing the risk of thrombosis is to address the pathological risk factors (e.g. diabetes, obesity). However, in practice, this is often difficult (e.g. surgery), and we fall back on medicines. Although clotting involves platelet activation, VTE prevention and treatment is generally aimed at clotting proteins like fibrinogen. There are two families of drugs: oral (the VKA antagonists (principally warfarin) and the NOACs) and parenteral (heparins and hirudins). However, there are also some non-drug treatments. A key reference book for all drugs is the British National Formulary (BNF). This important book (also available free on-line) not only lists drugs, but also gives indications, doses and hazards such as the effects of other drugs.

Vitamin K antagonists (VKAs)

Vitamin K, normally obtained in our diet, is an essential requirement in our ability to synthesise key molecules involved in coagulation, so if we are deficient in this vitamin (such as by diet), we can't make them as well and so don't clot that efficiently. There are several drugs in this class.

Warfarin

This is traditionally the most widely used anticoagulant in the UK and western world. It is a slow poison that specifically blocks the liver's production of vitamin K-dependent prothrombin and Factors VII and X, protein C and protein S. Thus, in the laboratory and in the body, clotting takes longer to happen. This leads, in real terms, to a protection from inappropriate thrombosis.

Use of warfarin demands frequent laboratory monitoring. The patient's **prothrombin time (PT)** is compared to normal plasma, to produce the **International Normalised Ratio (INR)**. The degree of anticoagulation required depends on clinical circumstance but target INR usually ranges from 2 to 4. Because warfarin has a narrow therapeutic index, changes in health or concurrent medication require more intensive monitoring of the INR.

The INR is simply the ratio between the times that whole blood or plasma (i.e. the prothrombin time) takes to clot normally, compared to the (supposedly increased) time it takes to clot due to warfarin. We use the INR to strike a balance between slowing down the clot-forming process, and the use of too much warfarin, which will interfere with clotting so much that a clot may never happen.

Phenidione and acenocoumarol

These are alternative oral vitamin K antagonists for those unwilling or unable to tolerate warfarin. However, concerns regarding the potential for hepatotoxicity, nephrotoxicity and other blood problems have reduced its role largely to those allergic to, intolerant of, or hypersensitive to warfarin.

NOACs

These non-vitamin K antagonist oral anticoagulants represent a major step forward in anticoagulation. Unlike the VKAs, NOACs act directly on certain molecules of the coagulation pathway. One of the consequences of this is that they are markedly more efficient than the indirect VKAs. A further advantage is that (like LMWH) they do not need a routine blood test, and have a much better safety profile, although there may always be non-specific side effects. In addition, some NOACs are more efficient than the traditional drug (in terms of reductions in VTE and stroke), and are also (generally) safer, in that there are fewer cases of haemorrhage. NOACs can be classified by the particular coagulation molecule they inhibit.

Direct thrombin inhibitors

The only oral **direct thrombin inhibitor** is **dabigatran**. It has been licensed in Europe for the prevention of stroke and VTE in atrial fibrillation, and for the prevention of VTE following orthopaedic surgery. It is likely that in due course it will be licensed for the treatment of acute VTE and prevention of recurrent VTE.

Factor Xa inhibitors

There are three **Factor Xa inhibitors**, all having the suffix '-xaban'. These are **rivaroxaban**, **apixaban** and **edoxaban**. However, not all of them have the same licences, although it is likely that eventually each of the NOACs will be licensed for the same indications.

Heparin

This natural anticoagulant's major effect is accounted for by its support for anti-thrombin in the (obvious) inactivation of thrombin but also coagulation Factor Xa (and some others). The short half-life means that it must be given continuously, and it must be given parenterally (through the skin), preferably by continuous IV infusion (i.e. a pump) and is therefore inappropriate for home use. The effect of heparin on the clotting cascade must be monitored in the laboratory by measuring the **activated partial thromboplastin time** (**APTT**), generally aiming for an **APTT ratio** of 1.5 to 2.5 times that of someone not on this drug. This system is a rough parallel to the use of the INR for warfarin treatment.

The proven efficacy of heparin in numerous settings (e.g. DVT, in acute coronary syndromes) must, like that of warfarin, be set against adverse effects. These include haemorrhage, osteoporosis, alopecia and hypersensitivity. However, probably the most important is a low platelet count, perhaps less than 100×10^9/L, and certainly less than 50×10^9/L, i.e. **thrombocytopenia**. Hence this **heparin-induced thrombocytopenia** (**HIT**), which happens in perhaps 1–3% of patients on this drug, can compound a bleeding event and even cause a thrombosis. If this happens then the heparin must be stopped and an alternative anticoagulant provided.

Heparin is available as a non-proprietary drug, but also as tradenames Calciparine, Monoparin, Monoparin calcium, and Multiparin. Structurally, 'old-fashioned' **unfractionated heparin** (so also known as **UFH**) is quite a crude preparation, being a mixture of numerous different types of sugary molecules; some fragments are smaller, others larger. About 20 years ago it was 'cleaned up' into a new preparation.

Low Molecular Weight Heparin (LMWH)

This is a much safer preparation of heparin. Although it also cannot be taken orally, it is safe enough to be given by one-off injection, even in out-patients and at home, and does not need to be monitored in the laboratory by the APTT test. A further good point is that there is also a reduced incidence of side effects such as osteoporosis and HIT. The differences between the old-style unfractionated heparin and the newer LMWHs are outlined in Table 4.1.

In those few cases where monitoring is deemed necessary (e.g. to test the effective dose in prophylaxis of VTE in high-risk pregnancy), laboratory measurement of plasma levels of anti-Factor Xa activity are required. Tests of APTT are unhelpful.

The British National Formulary (September 2014) lists three different types of LMWH:

● Dalteparin (Fragmin)

● Enoxaparin (Clexane)

● Tinzaparin (Innohep).

These preparations vary in the licences that they have been granted for use in different clinical conditions, but also in the ratio of anti-Xa to anti-thrombin activity, although the clinical relevance of this is uncertain. Also listed is the heparinoid called Danaparoid (Organan).

Table 4.1
Comparison of LMWH and unfractionated heparin

	Unfractionated heparin	LMWH
Action	Anti-thrombin, Factor Xa, and others	Almost completely anti-Xa
Route of administration	Subcutaneous or intravenous	Subcutaneous
Subcutaneous adsorption	Slow	Improved
Protein-binding	Proteins in plasma and on endothelium	Reduced protein binding so more effective
Approx mol. weight	15,000	4,000–6,000
Effective half-life	Subcutaneous: 1.5 hours Intravenous: 30 minutes	4 hours
Between and within individual variation	Extensive	Minimal
Monitoring	APPT	If required, anti-Xa activity
Elimination	Liver and kidney: so failure of both organs is important	Kidney: so renal function must be considered

Other anticoagulants

Fondaparinux

Fondaparinux is a selective and reversible Xa-inhibitor, and although based on the structure of heparin, it is different from both heparin and LMWH. Pharmacokinetics are characterised by a 100% bioavailability by subcutaneous route, lack of bio-metabolism, urinary excretion and a relatively long plasma half-life of 14–21 hours.

With a rapid onset of action, peak activity is reached in 2 hours. No interactions with aspirin, warfarin or digoxin have been noted.

Fondaparinux, like LMWHs, does not affect the prothrombin time (PT) and has very weak effects on the APPT. Its activity can be determined by specific anti-Xa assays, if necessary. Thrombocytopenia (platelet count <100 x 109/L) occurs even less frequently than with LMWH.

Hirudins

These small anticoagulant peptides, purified from the leech Hirudo medicinalis, bind thrombin with high specificity and sensitivity. With a true half-life of about an hour, hirudin has a half-life effect on the APTT of 2–3 hours. Consequently it may be seen as a competitor to heparin in several indications, such as HIT and unstable angina, etc. Brands include Hirulog, Argatroban, Desirudin, Lepirudin and Bivalirudin (see the BNF).

Dextran

This polysaccharide is cumbersome and may give rise to adverse effects, so is rarely used. See the BNF for additional details on all agents.

Non-drug treatments

General measures

As immobility increases the risk of DVT about ten-fold, early mobilisation and leg exercises to reduce stasis should be encouraged in all patients as much as is practicable. Similarly, as haemoconcentration increases blood viscosity and reduces blood flow, adequate hydration should be ensured in all patients.

Inferior vena cava filters

The key document in this section is the guideline on the use of vena cava filters (VCFs) published in the *British Journal of Haematology* (2006, 13: 590–5) by the British Committee for Standards in Haematology. See www.bschguidelines.com.

If (some say 'when') DVTs in the legs embolise and clots pass up the vena cava, they may ultimately end up in the lung and so cause a PE. One way to prevent formation of a PE is to physically prevent these small thrombi from reaching the lung by placing a filter in the inferior vena cava (hence VCF) often at a level just below the renal veins. From the technical point of view, VCFs are best placed with assistance from ultrasound and fluoroscopy, quite probably by an interventional radiologist. The use of VCFs focuses on:

- patients who have a contraindication to anticoagulation
- pregnant women who develop VTE shortly before delivery (whether or not they have a contraindication for anticoagulation)
- selected patients with PE despite therapeutic anticoagulation, although these patients may benefit from high dose warfarin (target INR 3.5) or LMWH prior to VCF placement, particularly in patients with thrombophilia or cancer.

VCFs are not indicated in unselected patients with VTE who receive conventional pharmacotherapy, in those undergoing thrombolysis, or in those with free-floating thrombus. However, it is common practice to initiate anticoagulation after VCF placement if and when there is no longer a contra-indication to anticoagulation. Although VCFs have been shown to reduce the occurrence of new PEs, curiously, they also bring a risk of new DVT. This happened despite the use of anticoagulant therapy. Early complications of VCF placement include insertion site thrombosis and infection. Late complications include recurrent DVT, inferior vena cava thrombosis and post-thrombotic syndrome.

Thus the decision to introduce anticoagulant therapy in a patient with a VCF should be based on the perceived underlying risk of the condition and the likelihood of anticoagulant therapy-based bleeding.

Mechanical methods

Graduated elastic compression stockings (GECS) are effective in prophylaxis of asymptomatic DVT and symptomatic PE in surgical patients (n.b. suspender belts are also available). GECS are available in above and below knee but the former are preferred for DVT prophylaxis. However, there can be problems with GECS and certainly not all patients can tolerate them (see Table 5.5 to follow).

Intermittent pneumatic compression (IPC) devices periodically compress the calf and/or thigh muscles with an inflation pressure of 35–40mmHg for about 10 seconds to a minute. They are generally applied immediately before or during surgery, are effective in prophylaxis of asymptomatic DVT in surgical patients, and are often subsequently replaced by GECS.

Other mechanical and surgical treatments (e.g. **embolectomy**) are usually reserved for massive life-threatening PE where drug treatments have failed or are contraindicated.

The geko device, which resembles a small wrist-watch, when attached to the leg delivers a small electrical charge to the tissues that results in increased venous blood flow. This, it could be argued, helps prevent the formation of a DVT. Accordingly, it has been received positively by NICE (Medical technology guidance MTG19, June 2014) as of potential value in those unable to use other therapies.

Thrombolytic therapy (getting rid of the clot)

Unlike heparins and warfarin (that antagonise extension and recurrence of thrombosis), thrombolytic agents (e.g. streptokinase, urokinase, alteplase, reteplase – collectively called tissue plasminogen activators, tPAs) actually lyse the thrombi. However, indications for this therapy are unclear. Recent guidelines do not recommend thrombolysis or thrombectomy for DVT unless there is danger of the limb being lost (i.e. amputated).

Notably, these drugs are also used to treat the symptoms of acute myocardial infarction – i.e. the chest pain that is presumed to be the result of a thrombus in one of the coronary arteries. In acute PE, these treatments (e.g. alteplase 50mg) are reserved for the most serious and unstable cases, where there is haemodynamic instability. Thrombolytic therapy infusion into the pulmonary artery (after clot disruption using a pigtail catheter manipulated within the pulmonary artery) has been reported. As discussed, a VCF may be considered.

Anti-platelet therapy

Almost all patients should be able to tolerate oral or parenteral anticoagulant, but for the few who cannot (for whatever reason), anti-platelet drugs **aspirin** and **clopidogrel** (Plavix) are an alternative. However, it is established that anti-platelet drugs are not as effective in reducing the risk of VTE as are anticoagulant drugs, and provide no protection from stroke in atrial fibrillation. Anti-platelet therapy is the leading choice for the treatment of arterial thrombosis.

Consolidation (see pages 82–85 for answers)

4.1 How does warfarin work?

4.2 How do we monitor the effect of warfarin on the blood?

4.3 Can you name any disadvantages of heparin?

4.4 Why are NOACs an advance on traditional drugs?

4.5 What non-drug treatments are available?

Case Study 2

A 69-year-old woman has elective hip-replacement surgery. Her recovery is good and she is maintained after her operation with analgesia and unfractionated heparin. However, on the day of her discharge a few days later, she starts to suffer nose-bleeds and her wound begins to ooze. A blood test for her heparin reveals an APTT ratio of 2.1 (desired result between 1.5 and 2.5) but a platelet count of 75 x 10⁹ cells/mL (desired range between 140 and 400).

What has happened and what do you need to do?

Chapter 5

Clinical practice of anticoagulation

These pharmaceutical agents can be dangerous and must be used with care – overuse can lead to life-terminating haemorrhage. However, there are numerous guidelines about how to use these drugs in different clinical settings. Many such guidelines are based on books and published research papers, many of which are available on the internet, and many are free.

- Perhaps the most accessible is the British National Formulary (BNF), widely available in NHS hospitals and regularly updated. See www.bnf.org.
- The British Committee for Standards in Haematology (BCSH) offers reasonably up-to-date guidelines for out-patient treatment of DVT with warfarin or heparin at www.bschguidelines.com.
- Powerful resources are provided by NICE (www.NICE.org.uk), which publishes clinical guidelines (CG) on the management of certain conditions, such as CGs 92, 144 and 180. A second set of publications appraises drugs such as the NOACs.

Local practice and management

The House of Commons Health committee report 'The Prevention of Venous Thrombo-embolism in Hospitalised Patients' (The Stationery Office 2005) recommends that each hospital establish a '**Thrombosis Committee**'. There is the clear implication that this committee will co-ordinate and issue local guidelines. As indicated above, NICE, the UK national guideline-setting body, releases numerous documents that demand attention. Another body, the **National Patient Safety Agency** (**NPSA**) has released its own guidelines on the management of the patient on warfarin.

A Trust or other body undertaking anticoagulation is required to set its own internal guidelines, based on documents such as those from NICE and the NPSA, which may not apply to another Trust, CCG, General Practice or, indeed, practitioner.

> **Therefore ...**
>
> what follows is informed comment and **NOT** guidelines.
>
> **NO** responsibility is taken for their use in clinical practice.
>
> Practitioners are expected to refer to their own local guidelines.

All patients admitted to an NHS hospital must be assessed for their risk of developing a VTE. Indeed, most in-patients (surgical or medical) are likely to be at a relatively high and acute risk of thrombosis, in which case they are likely to be treated with an anticoagulant such as a LMWH or a NOAC. However, it is also possible that some patients will come in to hospital already taking warfarin or a NOAC. If so, this may need to be reduced or stopped altogether. Patients, especially those undergoing surgery, may also benefit from GECS. In many cases the risk of thrombosis will still be present after the patient is fit for discharge. If so, the patient is likely to be discharged with GECS and treated with an oral anticoagulant (NOAC or VKA) as an out-patient. These will most likely be commenced on the ward.

Patients may also be referred for anticoagulation (perhaps by a Trust colleague or by a General Practitioner) whilst not at immediate acute risk of thrombosis (e.g. with newly diagnosed atrial fibrillation).

The text that follows will adopt this general scheme. The immediate clinical questions will be suggestions relevant to prophylaxis with LMWH or a NOAC in medical and surgical in-patients. These are preferred to VKAs, which have a long time to effectiveness, and so bring management problems. As in many cases the risk of thrombosis will extend beyond the patient's stay in hospital, then out-patient prophylaxis will become necessary. Comments regarding the use of oral anticoagulants (warfarin and NOACs) will therefore follow those for the use of LMWH.

Figure 5.1 illustrates these issues.

Risk assessment for treatment with LMWH

ALL in-patients (regardless of medical/surgical indication) **MUST** be assessed for the risk of developing VTE to identify those at highest risk and to identify any contra-indications to thromboprophylaxis. The practitioner will identify specific risk factors (introduced in Table 5.1), as some risk factors are more dangerous than others, and prepare a total score as follows.

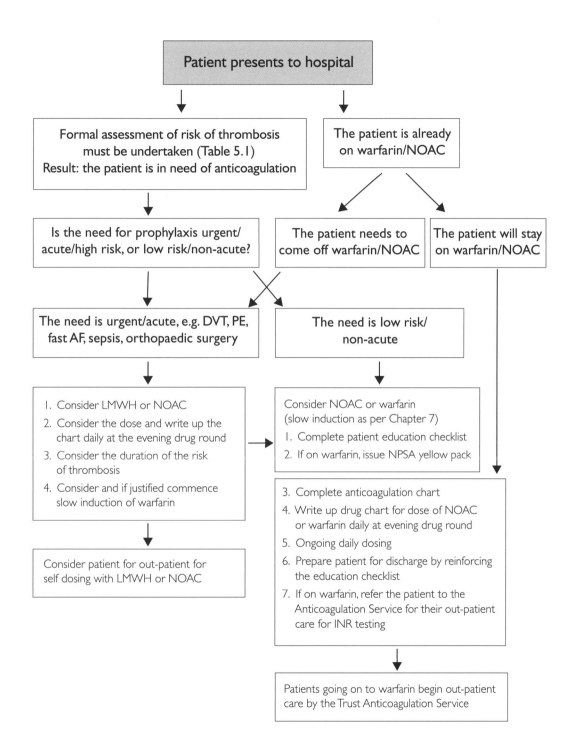

Figure 5.1 Anticoagulation management simplified

Table 5.1 Risk factors for VTE

Risk Factors (Score 1)	Risk Factors (Score 2)	Risk Factors (Score 3)
Age >60	Oestrogen-containing pill	Immobile (>72 hours)
Obesity (BMI >30)	HRT	History of DVT/PE
IHD, CCF or previous stroke	Known thrombophilic conditions	
Significant COPD	Malignancy	
Extensive varicose veins	Sepsis	
Inflammatory bowel disease or nephrotic syndrome	Known family history in 2 relatives (at least 1 first degree)	
Myeloproliferative disorders	Pregnancy and post-partum	

As with all tables, local guidelines take precedence

BMI = body mass index, IHD = ischaemic heart disease, CCF = congestive cardiac failure
HRT = hormone replacement therapy, COPD = Chronic obstructive pulmonary disease
(modified from NICE CG92)

For elective admissions for surgery an assessment of risk should take place at the pre-assessment clinic appointment, where appropriate. For all others, the assessment of risk should take place on admission to the ward. Where patients are undergoing surgery, high-risk procedures should be taken into consideration as some procedures are more likely to cause a DVT or PE than are others (Table 5.2).

Often, day surgery patients do not routinely receive anticoagulation, as they are mobile within a few hours postoperatively. However, it is possible that patients at risk of VTE may be admitted as a day case. The suitability of such patients for one dose of LMWH or NOAC should be discussed with the consultant in charge.

The total risk score will give an initial guide to therapy, although LMWH or a NOAC may not be appropriate for all patients. If so, anti-platelet therapy (aspirin *and/or* clopidogrel) is an option.

Contra-indications to anticoagulation

After clinical assessment has demonstrated an indication for anticoagulant prophylaxis, the patient's medical and drug history must be assessed for the cautions and contra-indications to particular agents. These are indicated in Tables 5.3 and 5.4.

Table 5.2 Additional risk factors for surgical in-patients

Score	Surgical Procedure
4	Major trauma, e.g. lower limb fractures
4	Major joint replacement
4	Surgery for fractured neck of femur
3	Thoracotomy or abdominal surgery involving mid-line laparotomy
3	Total abdominal hysterectomy, including laparoscopic assisted
2	Intraperitoneal laparoscopic surgery lasting >30 minutes
2	Vascular surgery (not intra-abdominal)
I	Surgery lasting >30 minutes
0	Surgery lasting <30 minutes

As with all tables, local guidelines take precedence

Table 5.3 Contra-indications and cautions to heparin prophylaxis

Contra-indications	Cautions
Known uncorrected bleeding disorders, e.g. haemophilias	Severe hepatic impairment
Severe to moderate thrombocytopenia (seek advice)	Severe renal impairment
Heparin allergy	Major trauma or surgery to the brain, eye or spinal cord.
Heparin-induced thrombocytopenia	
Heparin-induced thrombosis	
Patients on existing anticoagulation therapy	
Bleeding or potentially bleeding lesions, e.g.	
● Oesophageal varices, active peptic ulcer	
● Recent intracranial haemorrhage	
● Intracranial aneurysm or vascular malformation	

As with all tables, local guidelines take precedence

Table 5.4 Contra-indications and cautions to OAC prophylaxis

Contra-indications	Cautions
Peptic ulcer	Recent surgery
Severe hypertension (BP >160/100)	Alcohol abuse
Thrombocytopenia (platelet count <100)	Previous haemorrhage
Bacterial endocarditis	Dementia
(For NOACs, severe renal failure)	Hepatic impairment (raised LFTs)
	Moderate renal impairment
	Breast feeding

As with all tables, local guidelines take precedence

In addition, pregnancy is a contra-indication for VKAs. Indeed, women of child-bearing age taking warfarin should be made aware of the risk of teratogenicity. The drinking of cranberry juice on a VKA should be prohibited (see also the latest version of the BNF).

It follows that for some patients, anticoagulation will not be appropriate. In which case, an alternative is required if the risk of thrombosis is to be reduced. The issues of safety will be recapitulated wherever necessary.

Non-pharmacological treatments

All in-patients will be considered for the use of graduated elastic compression stockings (GECS) (see page 20). However, contra-indications and cautions apply. The practitioner will consider these before recommending their use (Table 5.5).

GECS may be full length, thigh length, or below-knee. Most clinically important DVTs occur above the knee, which provides the rationale for using full-length stockings. Most controlled studies have used above-knee stockings and the trials comparing above-knee and below-knee stockings have been too small to determine whether or not they are equally effective. This must be balanced against the evidence, which suggests that below-knee stockings are better tolerated by patients and easier to apply. All GECS should be prescribed on the drug chart.

The in-patient will be mobilised as much as is practicable, and full attention will be given to adequate hydration.

Table 5.5 Contra-indications and cautions for the use of GECS

Contra-indications	Cautions
Massive oedema of the legs or pulmonary oedema from congestive heart failure	Select correct size. Apply carefully, aligning toe hole under toe
Severe arteriosclerosis or other vascular disease of the leg	Check fitting daily for change in leg circumference
Extreme deformity of the leg	Do not fold down
Local leg condition, e.g. dermatitis, gangrene	Remove daily for no more than 30 minutes

As with all tables, local guidelines take precedence

Treatment

Once:

(a) the patient has been assessed and found to be in need of treatment, and

(b) the contra-indications or cautions to anticoagulation have been addressed

then:

(c) the patient must be informed and educated as to the purpose of the particular treatment, and

(d) treatment can begin according to the following regimes.

1. Acute risk of VTE and no contra-indications for LMWH/NOAC

The process calls for a sum of scores for risk factors (Table 5.1) and surgical procedures (Table 5.2) into an overall score (Table 5.6). Notably, almost all patients will score at least 2, more if undergoing surgery, and therefore inevitably will be in need of anticoagulation. Because the risk is acute, warfarin cannot be used (it requires several days to become effective).

Table 5.6
Application of risk assessment tables for the use of LMWH/NOAC

Low Risk – Score 0 or 1	Moderate Risk – Score 2 or 3	High Risk – Score 4
Early ambulation Consider GECS	GECS Low dose LMWH od for surgical patients High dose LMWH od for medical patients A NOAC	GECS High dose LMWH od (max. 14 days for medical in-patients) Surgical patients: consider IPC in theatre plus high dose LMWH A NOAC

Note: For male patients <57kg and female patients <45kg, caution may be needed regarding the dose of LMWH or NOAC prescribed. Renal function will also need to be checked as this will influence the dose of NOACs. Consult the clinician in charge of patient's care or local guidelines. IPC = intermittent pneumatic compression.

How much of the drug should be given?

For LMWH, this depends on a number of factors. First, the different varieties of LMWH all have different licences for different conditions, such as treatment of proven VTE, or the prevention of VTE that may arise from certain risky situations like orthopaedic surgery (i.e. prophylaxis). LMWHs have different potencies so that the dose from one may be different to the dose from another. Some suggest doses of a certain number of mg; other doses are for a given number of units. Secondly, it may also be the case that doses are different for those in need of treatment of an actual DVT or PE, or in prevention of a possible VTE that may occur in the near future (i.e. prophylaxis after a high-risk procedure such as hip replacement).

Although there are three NOACs (with one more in the pipeline), not all of them have NICE licences for all indications. As of September 2014, only rivaroxaban is licensed for the treatment and prevention of 'uncomplicated' DVT and PE (i.e. occurring without a likely cause such as orthopaedic surgery), and is available in different strengths (10mg, 15mg, 20mg) to enable a more effective anticoagulation for a short period, and to address renal failure. It is likely that other NOACs will also be licensed for these indications.

Prevention (prophylaxis) of VTE

The BNF (the latest issue of which must be consulted) recommends the dose of a particular LMWH for the prophylaxis of DVT in low-risk surgical patients to be 20mg (2000 units) 2 hours before surgery, then 20mg every following 24 hours for 7–10 days. A high-risk patient by the same token needs 40mg (4000 units) 12 hours before surgery and additional 40mg doses every 24 hours for 7–10 days. However, for medical patients, the dose is 40mg every 24 hours for at least 6 days and until ambulant, to a maximum of 14 days. NICE licenses rivaroxaban for the prevention of recurrent DVT and PE (TA287), whilst the closely related TA261 recommends the drug as an option for preventing recurrent DVT and PE after a diagnosis of acute DVT. The dose for preventing a VTE after orthopaedic surgery is 10mg once daily for 2–5 weeks. See also NICE CGs 92 and 144.

Treatment of VTE

However, the same BNF recommends a dose of 1.5mg/kg (150 units/kg) of the same LMWH every 24 hours for the treatment of a proven DVT/PE for at least 5 days and until adequate oral anticoagulation has been established. So an 80kg patient may receive 20mg for prevention, but six times as much (80 x 1.5 = 120mg) for treatment. At the practical level, this degree of treatment is likely to be of a newly acquired VTE, often in hospital and therefore as an in-patient. Other LMWHs may have a different dosing regime. NICE TA287 licenses rivaroxaban for the treatment of DVT and

PE whilst TA261 recommends rivaroxaban as an option for treating DVT after a diagnosis of acute DVT. It should be given initially as 15mg twice daily for 21 days, then 20mg once daily. However, the BNF has guidance regarding a reduced dose in renal failure. See also NICE CGs 9 and 144.

Pregnancy

Here there is a recommendation (although unlicensed) to weight-adjust the dose of LMWH used for treatment of VTE: for weight under 50kg use 40mg (4000 units) twice daily, for 50–70kg use 60mg (6000 units), for 70–90kg use 80mg (8000 units) and for over 90kg, use 100mg (10,000 units) – all twice daily. The manufacturer of rivaroxaban recommends it be avoided in pregnancy.

General points

Note that doses of some LMWHs and NOACs may need to be adjusted according to factors such as the weight, body mass index, and renal function (e.g. increased serum creatinine or reduced glomerular filtration rate). Some guidelines may recommend that the dose of LMWH should be that which inhibits Factor Xa to a certain level (i.e. anti-Factor Xa activity). However, other LMWHs may not need to be dosed to this level of precision, and may be given at a standard dose.

It is clear that the role of the Trust's Thrombosis Committee is to guide all hospital-based practitioners on whichever agent (type of LMWH or NOAC) best suits their individual requirements. Those in primary care are likely to refer to guidelines from their local hospital. Therefore the practitioner must consult their local guidelines, and recall that these may change from workplace to workplace.

2. Acute risk of VTE but contra-indications for LMWH/NOAC

If a LMWH or a NOAC is (very rarely) inappropriate then anti-platelet therapy (e.g. enteric coated aspirin 75–300mg od or clopidogrel 75mg od) may be considered. Commencement on warfarin may also be considered. However, contra-indications to aspirin exist, principally known allergy and gastric erosions.

3. Chronic risk of VTE

As we have seen from Table 2.1, there are several long-term conditions that bring a risk of VTE. Those that bring the highest risk include chronic heart failure, cancer, and disease of the valves of the heart (including artificial valves). The increased risk of VTE brought on by obesity in itself is not thought worthy of anticoagulation. However, in combination with other risk factors, anticoagulation may be justified.

Although we are focusing on VTE, in some conditions, such as chronic heart failure, mechanical prosthetic heart valves and atrial fibrillation (AF), the patient is at a greater risk of stroke. Although these may be seen as diseases of arteries, where anti-platelet drugs are effective, the risk of stroke is reduced further by anticoagulation. However, in lone chronic heart failure (i.e. with no other risk factors), either aspirin or warfarin may be used.

As daily injections with LMWH (possibly for life) are unacceptable, VKAs and NOACs are used for long-term treatment and prevention of VTE. Both oral agents have been trialled in the prevention of stroke and systemic embolism in AF, and broadly speaking, the latter are at least as effective as warfarin, sometimes more so. NOACs also have a superior safety profile to that of warfarin in terms of reduced haemorrhage. The uses of these agents in AF, orthopaedic surgery and VTE prophylaxis and treatment are addressed in more detail in Chapter 8, where NICE CG180 is essential.

Consolidation (see pages 82–85 for answers)

5.1 Which single document provides details about all anticoagulants?

5.2 What Trust body within your particular workplace should be consulted about best practice?

5.3 What is the basis of the risk factor method for providing treatment?

5.4 Are there patients who should not be given LMWH?

5.5 What are the options for the long-term treatment and prevention of VTE?

Chapter 6

Use of LMWH

1 General medicine

Most cases of VTE are triggered by causes other than surgery and most fatal PEs occur in medical patients. This group may include patients with:

- central venous lines, malignancy (greater if on chemotherapy)
- congestive heart or respiratory failure (including pneumonia)
- HRT, use of oral contraceptives, paralytic stroke
- post-partum, previous VTE, thrombophilia, bed rest >3 days
- immobility due to sitting (e.g. prolonged car or air travel, wheelchair)
- increasing age, obesity, pregnancy, varicose veins…… (i.e. Table 5.1).

The following pathway is to be followed in each newly admitted patient:

- There must be an assessment to decide whether or not thromboprophylaxis is indicated (Table 5.1).
- If it has been decided that LMWH is the treatment of choice (as opposed to a NOAC), the patient must be assessed for contra-indications to LMWH (Table 5.3) and to GECS (Table 5.5).
- If appropriate, the patient will then be treated and administered with LMWH as follows (Table 5.6):

Low-risk patients   – Early mobilisation
                               – Attention to hydration
                               – Consider GECS.

Moderate/High-risk patients   – Early mobilisation
                                         – Attention to hydration
                                         – LMWH s/c daily at 18:00
                                         – GECS.

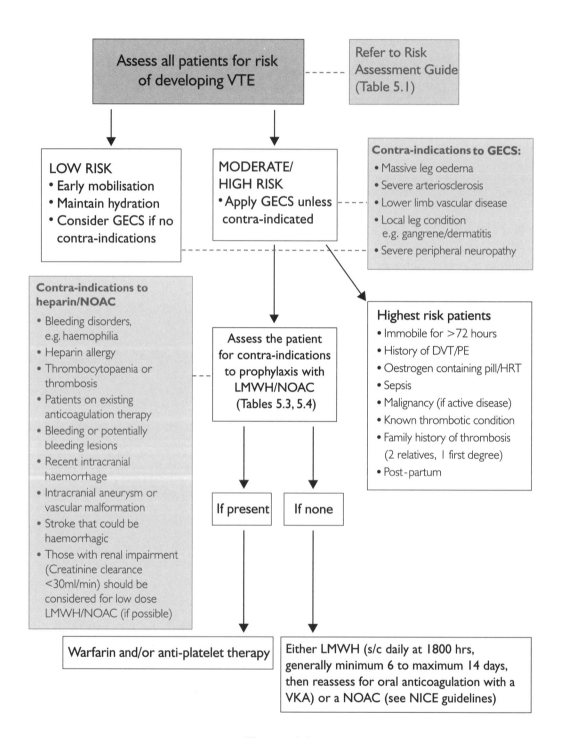

Figure 6.1
Algorithm for general medicine

Those patients intolerant of LMWH will need an alternative such as warfarin (probably target INR 2–3), aspirin (75–300mg daily) and/or clopidogrel (75mg daily) in addition to GECS. An alternative is a NOAC. Note that anti-platelet drugs are regarded as a treatment of last resort only in those patients unable to take anticoagulant drugs. Notably, this is the reverse of the treatment and prevention of arterial thrombosis (heart attack and stroke) where anti-platelet drugs are far more effective than anticoagulant drugs. Mechanical methods of prophylaxis have not to date been appropriately evaluated in acutely ill medical patients, and thus are not recommended at present.

All information will be recorded in the patient's medical notes.

Figure 6.1 summarises the use of LMWH in general medicine.

2 Acute cardiovascular emergencies

The two conditions under this umbrella are post-myocardial infarction (acute coronary syndrome) and cerebrovascular event (CVA, stroke). The former is specifically under the care of a cardiologist and more specific guidelines will apply. Similarly, treatment of acute stroke will also be under the close control of stroke physicians who will have their own guidelines. Practitioners are therefore likely to be involved in the anticoagulation of these groups under close scrutiny and closely structured guidelines.

Acute coronary syndrome (ACS)

In the initial management (e.g. in A&E, CCU) patients with an ACS are likely (in the absence of contra-indications) to be given aspirin 300–600mg followed by 150mg daily and are also likely to have clopidogrel 75mg daily after a loading dose of 300mg. Weight-adjusted LMWH (12 hourly) is started ASAP after initial assessment and continued for 3 days (and at least 24 hours after last documented ischaemic episode). For high-risk patients other anti-platelet drugs may be indicated (prasugrel, ticagrelor). As before, contra-indications include abnormal bleeding or stroke within 30 days, haemorrhagic stroke at any time, intracranial disease, severe hypertension (>160/110), increased PT, APTT, or thrombocytopenia.

For subsequent management (inevitably in CCU), cardiologists are likely to consider early coronary angiography (during the same admission) in patients who are candidates for revascularisation. Those with refractory symptoms, post-infarction angina, haemodynamic or rhythm instability require angiography as soon as possible. LMWH is likely to be omitted for at least 8–12 hours prior to angiography if planned.

If percutaneous coronary intervention (PCI) angiography demonstrates that angioplasty with possible stenting is appropriate, the procedure should ideally be carried out immediately (in the same session) if feasible, providing the patient is fully informed of the potential risk/benefit, or as soon as possible during the same admission. Patients undergoing PCI are likely to receive a reduced dose weight-adjusted bolus of UFH (30–70u/kg) as well as other drugs so that no further heparin should be given following the procedure (unless specified by the operator). All patients receiving coronary stents should also receive clopidogrel 300mg (if not already started) ASAP following the procedure, followed by 75mg daily for a minimum of 4 weeks (in addition to aspirin 75mg od). As of September 2014, there is no place for NOACs in the treatment of ACS, although this may change.

Stroke

The two different types of stroke each demand a completely different approach. Clearly, the haemorrhagic stroke is all about the patient having had a bleed into their brain, so the approach will be to minimise this bleeding. One method undergoing clinical trials is to provide an infusion of coagulation Factor VII to help the formation of a thrombus that aims to prevent the bleed getting worse.

In the alternative, a thrombotic stroke, the emphasis is on removing the clot and so starting revascularisation (as in an acute myocardial infarction). This may be possible by infusion of a tissue plasminogen activator (such as alteplase, NICE guidance, June 2007) to help dissolve the clot. An alternative is to try to remove the clot with a special catheter. Post-stroke, it may be necessary to use anticoagulation to reduce the risk of an additional thrombosis, alongside addressing the risk factors for VTE. As of September 2014, there is no place for NOACs in the treatment of stroke, although this may change. However, if the patient with AF has a history of stroke, a VKA or a NOAC is preferred over anti-platelets (NICE CG 180).

3 Surgery

N.b. NICE Guideline 92 applies

Traditionally, LMWH followed by a VKA (inevitably warfarin) has been the only option for preventing VTE after surgery. However, this view is fading in view of the advent of the NOACs. In this respect, NICE clinical guideline 46 (April 2007) has been replaced by clinical guideline 92 (January 2010), with the option to use dabigatran or rivaroxaban in certain types of orthopaedic surgery. The same guideline refers to an update due in July 2014, which is likely to refer to the use of apixaban in orthopaedic surgery, as currently recommended in NICE technology appraisal 245.

With the exception of those about to undergo orthopaedic surgery, almost all patients will qualify for prophylaxis with low dose LMWH od at 1800 hrs the evening before surgery unless prophylaxis is contra-indicated (see Table 5.3) and the patient has been identified as at highest risk of developing VTE. In this case a dose of high dose LMWH od at 1800 hrs should be prescribed (Figure 6.2).

Numerous bodies state that aspirin alone is not recommended for surgical patients as the only anti-thrombotic. Clearly, if the patient is intolerant of LMWH then anti-platelets, a NOAC or warfarin are the remaining options.

It is presumed that for elective surgery there has been full laboratory work-up with FBC, U&Es, LFTs etc. If the patient is already on warfarin or a NOAC, refer to Chapters 7 and 8 respectively.

A) Patients admitted the day(s) before surgery (Figure 6.2)

Whenever possible, prophylaxis with a high dose of LMWH should be commenced at 1800 hrs on the evening before surgery. This will achieve effective prophylaxis combined with minimal additional risk of bleeding complications at the time of regional anaesthesia (e.g. epidural or spinal) and surgery. Thereafter, low dose LMWH (more if at highest risk) should be continued at 1800 hrs daily at the same time until anticoagulation with warfarin has reached its target INR, or (in the case of minimal surgery in the young) until the risk of thromboembolism is considered to be minimal.

For patients undergoing Transurethral Resection of Prostate (TURP), low dose LMWH should be given on the evening before surgery (e.g. 1800 hrs) unless contra-indicated. Post-operative doses should be given as moderate or high risk as normal.

B) Patients admitted on the day of surgery

Patients eligible for prophylaxis should ideally receive a low dose of LMWH two hours pre-operatively, unless this is contra-indicated. One of the main contra-indications is that the patient is due to be receiving regional anaesthesia (spinal or epidural). See section D below.

Therefore, if a general anaesthetic only is to be administered, the pre-operative dose should be prescribed by the anaesthetist following the assessment. Patients should then receive a further low dose of LMWH at 1800 hrs on the evening following the surgery; for elective admission of those who have attended pre-operative assessment, this should have been already prescribed at the clinic.

Thereafter a daily low dose of LMWH at 1800 hrs should be prescribed, unless the patient is identified at highest risk, when high dose LMWH should be given.

C) Emergency patients

Patients admitted, who are eligible for prophylaxis and who are expected to be operated on within 12 hrs, should be treated as elective patients admitted on the day of surgery. Naturally, full blood work-up will need to be achieved ASAP as if on-call.

Patents who are admitted after 0900 hrs but who are not expected to be operated on until the following day should receive the recommended dose at 1800 hrs on the evening of admission.

In all cases

For the purposes of these notes, for surgical patients it is recommended that:

- LMWH prophylaxis should be continued at the same times daily until discharge or until the risk of thromboembolism is considered minimal (the latter most unlikely). However…
- Consideration should be given to extending prophylaxis when the hospital stay is prolonged or the risk continues. Such prophylaxis is likely to be with warfarin. An alternative is for out-patient treatment or the patient to self-dose with LMWH.
- Continued use of GECS on discharge from hospital to reduce the risk of late VTE may be beneficial in patients with poor mobility.
- NICE recommends that LMWH or fondaparinux therapy should be continued for 4 weeks after hip fracture surgery.

D) Regional anaesthesia

A major caution is that when epidural/spinal anaesthesia or spinal puncture is employed, patients anticoagulated or scheduled to be anticoagulated with heparin for the prevention of VTE are at risk of developing an epidural or spinal haematoma, which can result in long-term neurological dysfunction.

It is recommended that if LMWH has been administered pre-operatively, a period of 12 hours should elapse – but this may vary with different Trust Guidelines.

Whenever possible, elective surgical admissions should be identified for spinal anaesthesia at the pre-assessment clinic and admitted the day before surgery. They should then receive a high dose of LMWH at 1800 hrs. This will achieve effective prophylaxis combined with minimal additional risk of bleeding complications at the time of regional anaesthesia (e.g. epidural or spinal) and surgery.

In all other cases where the patient has been identified to receive regional anaesthesia, the pre-operative dose of prophylaxis should be withheld. Chemoprophylaxis should then start post-operatively. LMWH should be given no sooner than 4 hrs after neural block.

For elective surgical admissions who have attended for pre-assessment, the maintenance dose of LMWH should already have been prescribed for 1800 hrs. Therefore, the anaesthetist must give a written instruction not to administer the LMWH dose at 1800 hrs if contra-indicated.

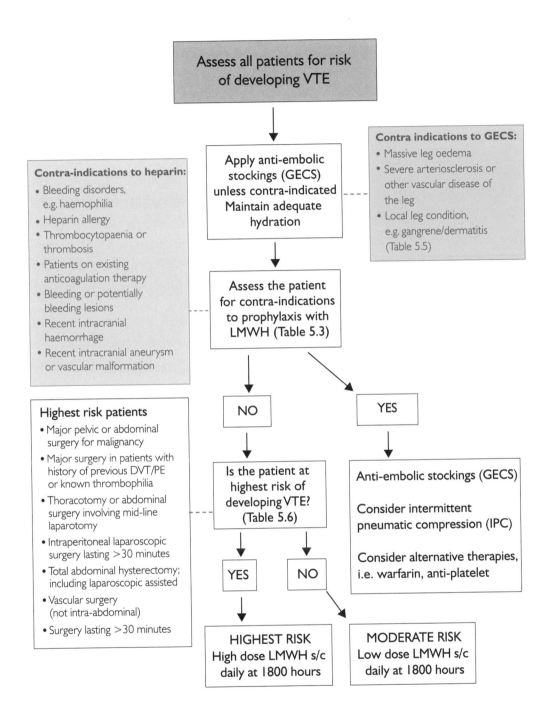

Figure 6.2
General algorithm for the use of LMWH in non-orthopaedic surgical patients admitted the day before their operation

4 Obstetric surgery (in cases of Caesarean section)

As yet there is no place for a NOAC in obstetric surgery, although they may be considered on a named-patient basis if all other anticoagulants are contra-indicated.

Elective Caesarean sections admitted the night before surgery
(see Figure 6.3)

In the case of planned Caesarean sections that are admitted the night before, low-dose LMWH should be started at 1800 hrs the evening before surgery, or if the woman is considered to be at high risk, a high dose of LMWH should be considered following discussion with the consultant responsible for her care. Thereafter, a dose of LMWH (dose dependent on risk) at 1800 hrs should be prescribed. Where epidural or spinal anaesthetic has been administered, the post-op day dose should be given no sooner than 4 hrs after spinal/epidural puncture.

Elective Caesarean sections admitted on the day of surgery
(see Figure 6.3)

Administer low-dose LMWH post-operatively on the day of surgery, provided that this is not within 4 hours if spinal or epidural anaesthesia has been administered (see section D above). Thereafter, low-dose LMWH od at 1800 hrs commencing the next day.

For the purposes of this guideline, for surgical patients it is recommended that:

● Heparin prophylaxis should be continued at the same times daily until discharge or until the risk of thromboembolism is considered minimal.
● Consideration should be given to extending prophylaxis when the hospital stay is prolonged or the risk continues. Such prophylaxis is likely to be with warfarin.
● Continued use of GECS on discharge from hospital to reduce the risk of late VTE may be beneficial in patients with poor mobility.

Oral contraceptives and hormone replacement therapy (HRT)

By themselves, the oral contraceptive pill and HRT are risk factors for VTE, as is surgery. It follows that women taking these synthetic hormones may be at additional risk of VTE should they continue this therapy during surgery. Certainly, such women on HRT undergoing surgery must be assessed for their risk of thrombosis, but there is no evidence in favour of routinely stopping HRT so long as there is appropriate thromboprophylaxis with LMWH or UFH. Recall that obesity and being bed-ridden are risk factors for VTE.

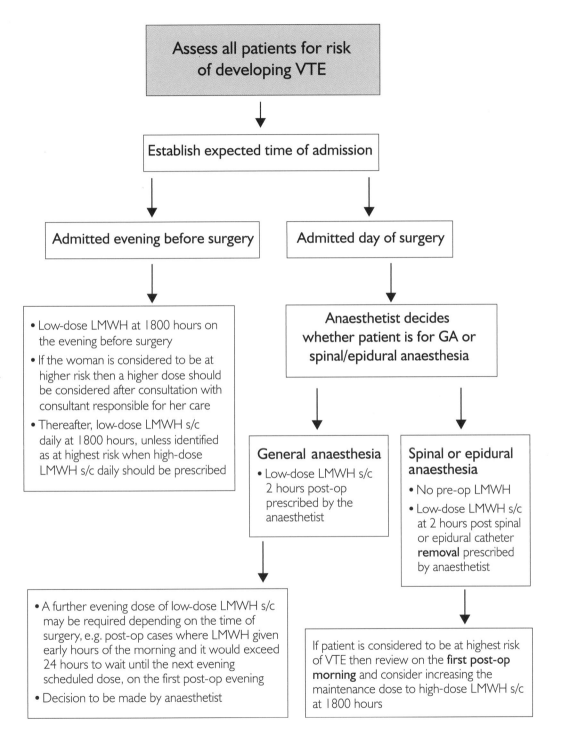

Figure 6.3 Guidelines for Caesarean section

Similarly, there is no evidence that the progesterone-only pill is associated with increased risk of VTE, or that such preparations should be stopped prior to surgery. However, whether or not to stop the combined (oestrogen plus progesterone) pill before major surgery is a controversial issue. The risk of unwanted pregnancy, the effects of anaesthesia on pregnancy and the risks of subsequent termination are high, and therefore, rather than stopping the OCP, these women should receive thromboprophylaxis with LMWH as per standard guidelines.

Consolidation (see pages 82–85 for answers)

6.1 What 'medical' patients may be in need of anticoagulation?

6.2 Which patient group should be given aspirin?

6.3 What is the most common time of day to give the patient their LMWH?

6.4 What is the role of the anaesthetist in providing anticoagulant cover?

6.5 What are the alternatives to LMWH?

Case Study 3

A 14-week pregnant woman, with a history of VTE (previous VTE at 38 weeks of pregnancy) and known to be heterozygous for FVL self-doses herself with 20mg of a LMWH daily. At routine screening, her anti-Factor Xa level is 0.5 units/mL (preferred therapeutic range 0.5–1.0, target prophylactic range 0.1–0.3 units/mL).

Do you take any action?

Chapter 7

Use of warfarin

General considerations

The National Patient Safety Agency (NPSA) alert 18

The document published by the NPSA refers predominantly to anti-thrombotic therapy as it is most frequently delivered by warfarin, although use of heparin is briefly addressed. In addition, its prescriptions are demanding, as action steps are strongly emphasised. These are:

- Ensure all staff caring for patients on anticoagulation therapy have the necessary work competencies. Any gaps in competence must be addressed through training to ensure that all staff may undertake their duties safely.

- Review, and, where necessary, update written procedures and clinical protocols to ensure they reflect safe practice, and that staff are trained in these procedures.

- Audit anticoagulant services using BSH (British Society for Haematology)/NPSA safety indicators as part of the annual medicines management audit programme. The audit results should inform local actions to improve the safe use of anticoagulants, and should be communicated to clinical governance, and drugs and therapeutics committees (or equivalents).

- Ensure that patients prescribed anticoagulants receive appropriate verbal and written information at the start of therapy, at hospital discharge, on the first anticoagulant clinic appointment, and when necessary throughout the course of their treatment.

- Promote safe practice with prescribers and pharmacists to check their patients' blood clotting (INR) is being monitored regularly and that the INR level is safe before issuing or dispensing repeat prescriptions for oral anticoagulants.

- Promote safe practice for prescribers co-prescribing one or more clinically significant interacting medicines for patients already on oral anticoagulants; to make arrangements for additional INR blood tests, and to inform the anticoagulant service that an interacting medicine has been prescribed.

- Ensure that dental practitioners manage patients on anticoagulants according to evidence-based therapeutic guidelines. In most cases, dental treatment should proceed as normal and oral anticoagulant treatment should not be stopped or the dosage be decreased inappropriately.

- Amend local policies to standardise the range of anticoagulant products used, incorporating characteristics identified by patients as promoting safer use.

- Promote the use of written safe practice procedures for the administration of anticoagulants in social care settings. It is safe practice for all dose changes to be confirmed in writing by the prescriber. A risk assessment should be undertaken on the use of Monitored Dosage Systems (MDS) for anticoagulants for individual patients. The general use of MDS for anticoagulants should be minimised, as dosage changes using these systems are more difficult.

- **Key reference: www.npsa.nhs.uk/health/alerts.**

The NPSA documents place considerable onus on Trust Thrombosis Teams and Committees to provide training for staff, education for patients, and guidelines for practitioners.

General notes

- These notes (and indeed, the entire book!) refer to adult patients on warfarin. In applying the general principles and recommendations within these notes, the healthcare professional will need to continue to apply medical and surgical knowledge and clinical judgement to the management of individual patients. These views may not be appropriate in all circumstances. Decisions to adopt any particular actions must be made by the practitioner in the light of available clinical and published resources.

- Practitioners will be aware that several, if not all, NOACs may be recommended as an alternative to warfarin. They may need to refer to local, national (e.g. British Committee for Standards in Haematology) and/or NICE guidelines. Full details of the NOACs are presented in Chapter 8.

Review of pathophysiology

Recall that warfarin is in fact a slow-acting specific liver poison and as such attention must be paid to adequate liver function (therefore need for LFTs). This is pertinent as this organ is also the site of production of many coagulation proteins. In practice this means that the full effect of a fixed dose of warfarin will not be evident for several days, possibly a week or more. Conversely, the liver will be slow to recover once the drug has been withdrawn. However, vitamin K can be given to promote the return of coagulation protein synthesis.

Warfarin is available in 0.5mg, 1mg, 3mg and 5mg tablets. Patients take a combination daily with an aim to maintain an INR either between 2 and 3 (hence target 2.5), or between 3 and 4 (hence target 3.5). In practice the average dose is 4–6mg daily. The INR is monitored with venous blood or by fingerprick. Management is by simple up or down titration followed by re-testing. In case of low INR (at either target), the patient is advised to increase their daily dose of warfarin, and vice versa for an INR above the desired range. Precise algorithms for these dose changes and return visits for rechecking are provided below.

Management

Patients may be classified as follows: (1) those presenting to hospital (e.g. for surgery) whilst already on warfarin, (2) those who have to be started on warfarin whilst an in-patient (e.g. following orthopaedic surgery), and (3) those naive to warfarin. The text that follows will address each group in turn.

1 The patient being admitted is already on warfarin

Therefore, by definition, the patient is already at risk of thrombosis. It is likely that the purpose of the hospital visit will increase this risk, and in almost all cases use of LMWH will be advised. The difficulty is therefore the extent to which warfarin must be reduced and re-introduced after the particular procedure that demanded in-patient attendance.

It is very likely that the patient's INR will change in accordance with hospital admission (i.e. effects of diet, mobility, other treatments) and in consequence their INR will need to be checked at least every 48 hours, possibility 24 hours. Common reasons for patients to be presenting are for surgery and for cardioversion of atrial fibrillation back to normal rhythm.

If the patient is admitted for surgery,

the risk of VTE from stopping warfarin needs to be balanced against the risks of bleeding during surgery. The following should be addressed:

- The option to stop warfarin therapy pre-operatively and perform the procedure when the INR has returned to safe levels; administer full-dose anticoagulation with LMWH; or administer prophylactic doses of LMWH.

- The individual's risk of bleeding will vary both with the type of surgery, and with the presence of other risk factors for bleeding. Most surgery can be safely performed when the INR falls to 1.5.

- Period of time for INR to fall: for patients in a therapeutic range of INR 2–3, it takes approximately 4 days after stopping warfarin for INR to reach 1.5; for patients with a therapeutic range INR 3–4 and the elderly this may be longer.

The patient is admitted for elective surgery

(i) Minor risk of VTE

For minor surgery an INR of <2 should be achieved. For very minor procedures, some surgeons may operate at INR 2.5. For an INR range 2–3: omit warfarin for 2 days. INR range 3–4: omit warfarin for 3–4 days. Re-start warfarin post-operatively on the day of surgery at the maintenance dose (occasionally a boost in the dose of warfarin will be required).

(ii) Medium risk of VTE

These will be patients on long-term anticoagulants for atrial fibrillation, cardiomyopathy, previous single episode of VTE more than three months ago, mural thrombus, rheumatic mitral valve disease, new model prosthetic aortic valves, tissue valves.

● Before surgery. Stop warfarin 4 days prior to surgery. If INR is still high, a small dose of vitamin K (0.5–1mg orally) may be given if necessary. Consider stopping anti-platelet drugs (aspirin, clopidogrel) 5–7 days before surgery. Give high dose LMWH sc at 18:00, at least 12 hours before operation. On the morning of surgery check that the INR is <1.5.

● After surgery. Continue high-dose LMWH od post-operatively as above. Re-start warfarin as soon as patient is able to take oral fluids. When INR >2 for 48 hours stop LMWH.

(iii) High risk of VTE

E.g. patients on long-term anticoagulants for prosthetic mitral valve, old model aortic prosthetic valves, recurrent VTE, anti-phospholipid syndrome, recent (within the last 3 months) VTE. Patients who have had VTE (especially PE within the last month) are considered very high risk. If surgery is urgent and there are risk factors for bleeding, IVC filters should be considered.

● Before surgery. Recall that the risk of haemorrhage is greater than the risk of recurrent VTE, providing sub-therapeutic INRs are limited to 1–2 days only. Generally, stop warfarin 4–5 days before surgery, and consider stopping anti-platelets 5–7 days before surgery. Admit 2 days prior to surgery, check INR on admission and daily. In some cases low-dose LMWH can be used when the INR is <2.0, with a prophylactic dose given the night prior to surgery. The interval between full-dose LMWH and surgery should be 24 hours; and 12 hours between prophylactic LMWH and surgery.

● Day of surgery. Check INR and APTT. If INR <1.8, proceed with operation, if INR >1.8, delay operation. A small dose of vitamin K, e.g. 0.5–1mg IV, will lower the INR. The onset of action of IV vitamin K is 6–8 hours and it may take 3 to 4 days for warfarin to work when re-started. LMWH will need to be continued post-op.

● After surgery. Re-start therapeutic low dose of LMWH 12 hours post-op. Monitoring should not be necessary, but if so this can be achieved with anti-Xa levels. Re-start warfarin at the usual dose on the evening of the operation or as soon as the patient is able to take oral fluids and provided there is no undue bleeding. Continue LMWH and warfarin until INR > 2.5 (this is usually 5–7 days). Monitor INR daily – however, be cautious in increasing the dose of warfarin too rapidly, recalling that warfarin is a slow-acting poison. For patients who are at a higher risk of bleeding, IV unfractionated heparin is preferable as it has a shorter duration of action than warfarin or LMWH, and is more rapidly reversible although monitoring by APTT is required.

The patient is admitted for emergency surgery

Again consider is it minor or major surgery – does the INR need to be lowered? (See above.) If INR is >2.0 and urgent reversal is required, stop anticoagulant therapy, take blood samples (INR, FBC, crossmatch, other tests if indicated). If there is sufficient time before surgery, give vitamin K 0.5mg IV slowly. This will lower the INR in roughly 6–8 hours. The patient may be refractory to warfarin for 3–4 days after but this can be covered with LMWH. Larger doses of IV vitamin K 5–10mg can be given if continued anticoagulation is not needed again. Check INR prior to surgery: if > 2.0 and surgery is urgent and there is no time for vitamin K to work, give fresh frozen plasma (FFP) 10–15ml/kg or prothrombin complex concentrates. Repeat INR after FFP and before surgery. When INR ≤ 2.0, proceed with operation.

Note that separate guidelines exist for management of in-patients who are over-anticoagulated. Re-start warfarin in the post-op period as above with regard to risks of thrombosis/ haemorrhage. Ensure the patient is fully educated as to the purpose of therapy.

The patient is admitted for cardioversion for atrial fibrillation (AF)

It is already established that AF is a risk factor for thrombotic stroke and therefore requires thromboprophylaxis, almost exclusively with warfarin (INR range 2–3). This should be indefinite (i.e. for life) as the chances of the heartbeat returning to (normal) sinus rhythm are remote in nature and thus the risk of stroke will be present for life. However, pharmacotherapy may be effective, but if this fails or is inappropriate, there is cardioversion.

This is effectively an attempt to shock the heart back to sinus rhythm with electricity. Unfortunately this procedure in itself can precipitate a stroke. This may be because of the effect of the cardioversion, although it may also result from the embolism of an existing intra-cardiac thrombus. In either case, the risk of this cardioversion-precipitated stroke can be reduced by anticoagulation.

A common regime is to ensure INR range 2–3 for several weeks both before and after cardioversion. Almost by definition, the patient will be on warfarin for weeks if not months before cardioversion; hence in practice it will simply be a matter of withdrawing the warfarin once sinus rhythm has been re-established (as proven by electrocardiogram).

In the autumn of 2014, data was published indicating that rivaroxaban is a viable alternative to warfarin in providing anticoagulant cover regarding cardioversion. Local guidelines may apply, and this may ultimately enter national and international guidelines.

2 The patient being admitted needs to be started on warfarin

The practitioner and their team must first decide if warfarin or a NOAC is the better option. What follows presumes that warfarin is the agent of choice.

Local guidelines should be developed by a multidisciplinary team to ensure a safe, effective and consistent approach to the management of adult patients in primary and secondary care receiving warfarin. Often, the prescribing information contained in published guidelines is issued on the understanding that it is the best practice from available resources at the time of issue. The latest recommendations from the British Committee for Standards in Haematology should be followed. Teams should also be aware of the latest NPSA patient safety alert already mentioned.

Each Trust's/PCT's documents must give advice to prescribers and other healthcare professionals on managing patients on warfarin, e.g. prescribing considerations, monitoring requirements and factors affecting warfarin therapy. The user is reminded of the importance of the patient's handheld record in the form of an anticoagulant therapy record booklet. Due to the inherent complexity associated with warfarin use, communication between teams involved in patient care is of utmost importance, particularly since very often patients are initiated in secondary care and managed in primary care.

Key points

- Ensure it is safe for the patient to take warfarin (Table 5.4)
- Establish diagnosis, target INR and duration of therapy (Table 7.1)
- Assess patient compliance; identify any problems that may indicate the patient will not comply with treatment and monitoring
- Baseline investigations: LFTs, FBC, APTT/PT, U&Es, creatinine
- Full medical history and medication history at start, then regularly
- Anticoagulant therapy record booklet supplied, completed, and patient taken through information systematically
- Ensure adequate communication between primary and secondary care.

Q: Who should be treated with warfarin?

A: Those in whom the benefits of warfarin outweigh the possible disadvantages.

Likely candidates for the prescription include those at risk of thrombosis (e.g. following orthopaedic surgery), but also those with a history of existing thrombosis (i.e. previous or current PE and/or DVT). As mentioned, a NOAC may be preferred in certain circumstances (Chapter 8).

Q: How long should treatment last?

A: As long as the risk factor remains active.

So for risk factors such as surgery or childbirth, treatment will not be for long. If the risk factor is cancer, this may be until cured. Patients with recurrent VTEs (i.e. who are thrombophilic) will also be long-term users. See Table 5.1.

Table 7.1
Target INRs and recommended duration of anticoagulation

Indication	INR target	Duration
Pulmonary embolus	2.5	6 months
Distal DVT due to temporary risk factors	2.5	3 months
Proximal DVT or DVT of unknown cause or those associated with ongoing risk factors	2.5	6 months
VTE associated with malignancy	2.5	6 months then review
Recurrence of VTE, NOT on warfarin	2.5	Long term
Recurrence of VTE, WHILST on warfarin	3.5	Long term
Atrial fibrillation	2.5	Long term
AF for cardioversion (CV)	2.75	4 weeks pre-CV min. 4 weeks post-CV
Cardiomyopathy	2.5	Long term
Mural thrombus	2.5	3 months
Rheumatic mitral valve disease	2.5	Long term
Mechanical prosthetic heart valves (Aortic)*	3.0	Long term
Mechanical prosthetic heart valves (Mitral)*	3.5	Long term
Antiphospholipid syndrome (VTE)	2.5	Long term
Antiphospholipid syndrome (arterial thrombosis)	3.5	Long term
Thrombophilias	Discuss with haematologist	

*According to BCSH guidelines, target INRs may vary depending on valve type; if unsure use generic target for valve location. Patients referred to the anticoagulant clinic will be assigned a target INR as per BCSH guidelines UNLESS reasonable evidence is given to the contrary. (N.b. it is likely that a NOAC would be prescribed for the same time period as warfarin.)

Induction of warfarin

SAFETY: As with heparins, not all patients will be able to take warfarin and all must be assessed (Table 5.4). The clinical, cognitive and social status of the patient should be assessed to ensure they are willing and able to take the drug as intended and attend for regular blood tests. Anticoagulation is contra-indicated in a number of situations where the risks of harm are likely to outweigh the benefits of treatment. Many contra-indications are relative rather than absolute. Absolute contra-indications to warfarin (and, as it happens, to NOACs) include potential bleeding lesions, active peptic ulcer, oesophageal varices, aneurysm and proliferative retinopathy, recent organ biopsy, etc. Relative contra-indications include history of GI bleeds, renal failure, alcoholism, mental impairment, thrombocytopenia (platelet count <50), liver failure, coagulation disorders, interacting drugs (in particular NSAIDs), poor concordance, poor attendance at clinic (Table 5.4).

General considerations

- There are two approaches to the induction of anticoagulation: slow or rapid. Slow induction can be initiated in out-patient anticoagulant clinics but may be considered in patients for imminent discharge. Referrals may be considered for rapid induction in the community. Patients will not be started on warfarin without:
- A comprehensive diagnosis (i.e. not simply 'DVT – please treat', but, for example, 'DVT secondary to prostatic cancer – please treat'). The desired target INR (generally 2.5 or 3.5 – if not, justify) (Table 7.1)
- The duration of treatment (3 months, 6 months, long term).
- For all patients:
- Take baseline blood samples (LFTs, FBC, APTT/PT, U&Es, creatinine), full medical history (any cautions or contra-indications, pregnancy) and full medication history (consider interactions, herbal and over the counter medicines).
- Record information on anticoagulation chart.
- Give patients/carers verbal and written information regarding their treatment, complete patient education checklist and insert in patients' records. The NPSA patient information packs are available from the pharmacy and are available in different languages.

Rapid induction

This is generally for patients at high and/or acute risk of VTE, and will be the dominant procedure for in-patients. Rapid anticoagulation should achieve the target INR within 5 days. Heparin and warfarin should be started together and heparin continued until the INR has been within range for two consecutive days. Subcutaneous heparin is usually the treatment of choice for VTE and acute coronary syndromes.

Where rapid induction of warfarin is required, follow the normogram (e.g. Table 7.2). Care should be taken for patients with a low body weight (less than 50kg), elderly patients, those with a low albumin, liver or heart disease, or multiple interacting medications. In such cases a lower loading dose, e.g. 5mg on day 1, should be used. In some cases slow induction should be considered.

REMEMBER: Warfarin requirements can vary immediately post-op and with heart and liver disease and in elderly patients – therefore use of smaller loading dose is suggested. Beware drug interactions and polypharmacy. *See BNF before prescribing new treatment.*

Patients who have recently commenced OAC therapy as in-patients will need their INR checking regularly, usually by venepuncture on alternate days within the first week. Once stabilised, frequency of INR checks can lengthen, but changes in interacting medications must be accompanied by more frequent checks.

As discussed, patients (especially undergoing surgery) may be started on LMWH and warfarin at the same time. However, this may be altered by the use of LMWH, especially for those who are self-dosing.

Table 7.2
Daily dose of warfarin to achieve rapid induction of INR 2–3

INR day 1 (before Rx)	Warfarin dose	INR day 2	Warfarin dose	INR day 3	Warfarin dose	INR day 4	Warfarin dose on day 4 and maintenance dose
<1.4	10mg	<1.4	10mg	<1.4	12mg	<1.4	15mg
		1.4–1.7	6mg	1.4–2.1	5mg	1.4	8mg
		1.8–3.8	1mg	2.2–2.5	4mg	1.5–1.7	7mg
		>3.9	none	2.6–2.9	3mg	1.8–1.9	6mg
				3.0–3.3	2mg	2.0–2.4	5mg
				3.4–3.5	1mg	2.5–3.2	4mg
				3.6–4.0	0.5mg	3.3–4.0	3mg
				> 4.5	None	4.1–4.5	Miss next dose then 2mg
						>4.5	Miss two doses then 1mg

NOTE: baseline INRs >1.4 please discuss with Haematology Consultant. For INRs >5 see the section on over-anticoagulation.

Slow induction

It follows that this route will be applicable (mostly) to out-patients.

Many patients diagnosed with AF are deemed to be of relatively low VTE risk (daily TIA/CVA rate no higher than 1/1000 per day). As the vast majority are from an ageing population, rapid introduction is neither warranted nor safe. In the latter regard, both advanced age and recent initiation are risk factors for major warfarin-related haemorrhage.

It must be borne in mind that many of these patients may already be on a number of other medications, including those with known potential for interaction with coumarin anticoagulants. This patient group may also have hepatic congestion arising out of congestive cardiac failure, with further pharmacodynamic implications. Some patients are also likely to have reduced renal reserve. Finally, it is important to establish from the patient's GP/Secondary Care Physician (often, but not always, a cardiologist) whether the patient should remain on anti-platelet therapy, e.g. aspirin/clopidogrel alongside oral anticoagulation.

The induction regimen of choice is determined by the baseline capillary INR and the presence or absence of various risk factors, e.g. age ≥70 yrs, CCF, relevant previous bleeding history (e.g. haematuria), polypharmacy (especially if ≥3 potential interactions), excessive alcohol intake, co-existent aspirin/clopidogrel, social isolation, etc. (there could be others in individual cases). Table 7.3 gives a typical scheme.

Table 7.3
Daily dose of warfarin to achieve slow induction of INR 2–3, e.g. as out-patients

Baseline INR	Risk Factors	Daily warfarin dose	Repeat INR
≤1.2	No	4mg	1 week
1.3–1.4	No	4mg	1 week
≤1.2	Yes	3mg	1 week
1.3–1.4	Yes	3mg	3 days

Subsequent dosing

Increase 0.5mg to 1mg daily until INR 2–3, return in 3–7 days depending on INR. If INR >3, then reduce dose accordingly. If baseline INR is >1.4, discuss with consultant haematologist. Further investigations may need to be undertaken prior to this patient receiving warfarin as an out-patient. For INR 3–4, adopt similar method but 1mg/day higher.

Re-starting patients on warfarin therapy

Patients who have stopped warfarin therapy (for example, due to surgery) will need re-inducting on warfarin depending on their reasons for anticoagulation. Usually, patients with simple AF may just need to re-start their warfarin on their usual dose (taking into consideration any changes in medication or general well-being). The risks of over-anticoagulation and bleeding associated with rapid induction should be considered. Patients with prosthetic valves may need anticoagulation cover with LMWH until INR is within range, depending on the age and valve type. Patients with a history of or recent VTE should receive LMWH until their INR is back within range. In both cases warfarin should be inducted rapidly. Consideration needs to be given post-operatively to increased risks of bleeding.

The Yellow Book

In the UK perhaps 500,000 people are taking warfarin, but with the advent of NOACs, this number will fall. A handy, if not invaluable, record of their treatment dose and INR is in the form of a Yellow Book that will be issued to each patient when they start on warfarin. It contains not only a record of the patient's warfarin use, but also helpful tips as to how the patients can help themselves, and what possible problems to be aware of. Patients are encouraged to take care of this book and bring it with them each time they attend hospital or their GP.

Generally

- Patients induced as in-patients will inevitably convert to out-patients.
- Some out-patients with special needs may need to be treated at home, i.e. they are 'domiciliary' patients.
- Many out-patients will be transferred to out-reach clinics, generally in GP surgeries, healthcare centres, etc.

Consolidation (see pages 82–85 for answers)

7.1 What government agency has published a major document on the general management of warfarin?

7.2 Why should patients about to undergo surgery be taken off warfarin and what is the alternative anticoagulant?

7.3 How long should treatment with warfarin last?

7.4 What kinds of patients require rapid induction or slow induction of warfarin?

3 On-going management of warfarin

All major teaching hospitals and District General Hospitals (DGHs) have an Oral Anticoagulant Therapy (OAT) Clinic, set up to serve possibly hundreds of patients taking (mostly) warfarin, although there is an alternative for those intolerant of this drug (phenidione). As discussed, warfarin is the most effective agent for reducing the risk of thrombosis, e.g. of thrombotic stroke in AF, and of a recurrent VTE, out-performing aspirin.

However, poor pharmacokinetics means it must be monitored frequently with a blood test (generally a thumb prick). Most hospitals provide this monitoring service for consultant colleagues or GPs, but once the INR has been checked it is logistically sensible to offer advice on management at the same time (i.e. on increasing or decreasing the daily dose of warfarin to be taken).

The objective of treatment with warfarin is to provide maximum reduction in risk of thrombosis with minimum risk of haemorrhage. For most patients, this is INR range 2–3. INR <1.6 (for example) provides low risk of haemorrhage but poor reduction in the risk of thrombosis. Similarly, a patient with INR 4.5 has superb protection against a thrombus but a high risk of bleeding.

Almost all literature deals with inappropriately high levels of INR, and mostly ignores a sub-therapeutic INR. However, many consider patients with a recent VTE to be at increased risk of recurrence, so that those with a sub-therapeutic INR of, shall we say, 1.2, on two concurrent visits, may need urgent LMWH (perhaps 20mg or 40mg) to minimise the risk of thrombosis until the INR is in its target range of 2–3.

Up- or down-titrate

At the practical level, a patient with an INR above target will be advised to cut down their daily dose, whilst those with an INR below range will be advised to increase their dose (i.e. up- or down-titration). Both sets of patients are then advised to return at an interval of 1–3 weeks (depending on history, risk factor profile, how far they are out of ideal target range).

Warfarin is offered in 0.5, 1, 3 and 5mg tablets, and the daily dose is made up by a combination. Cutting tablets in half is discouraged, so for 4.5mg a day, a patient will be instructed to take 4mg or 5mg on alternate days. But if, say, 4.5mg is too much, and 4mg too little, then 4.25mg seems correct. However, a daily or alternative day regime for this is impossible, but in practice, it may be achieved by taking 4mg each day, but 5mg on Wednesdays and Sundays, so that over the week it smooths out. Conversely, for a desired average dose of 3.75mg daily (where 4mg a day is too much but 3mg/4mg alternate days is not enough), a weekly regime would be 4mg a day but only 3mg on Wednesday and Sunday.

In one published study the typical daily dose of warfarin used by *low-risk* out-patients (i.e. INR target 2.5) was 4.5mg/day. Similarly, the typical daily dose used by *high-risk* out-patients (i.e. INR target 3.5) was 5.75mg/day.

Problems with management

Regrettably, as mentioned, the efficacy of warfarin is influenced by many factors that frustrate the objective of perfect INR control (Table 7.4). In practice, this means there is a considerable variability in its effect on patients, as its effectiveness is often influenced by factors such as age, racial background, diet and the use of other medications such as antibiotics. This will be revisited in due course.

Table 7.4
Patient factors that influence the efficacy of warfarin

Enhanced Anticoagulant Effect	Reduced Anticoagulant Effect
Excess alcohol ingestion	Weight gain
Increased age (e.g. >80 years)	Diarrhoea and vomiting
Heart and renal failure	Relative youth (e.g. age <40 years)
Impaired liver function	Non-White European background

Management options

A common model operates in two out-patient department rooms with a healthcare assistant, an occasional clerical assistant, a scientist, and a dosing officer (DO), all managed by a senior scientist with two full-time clerical assistants, and is heavily dependent on software. The clinic caters for around 100 patients three times a week who attend at regular intervals throughout a morning (9.30–12.30 pm) or afternoon (1.30–4.30 pm) session.

- Upon arrival, ideally at the rate of three per five minutes, patients are 'booked in' by a health-care assistant and queue up to have their blood checked. A clerical assistant is present for the first hour or so to sort out any administrative problems, such as lost details or new patients.

- In one room, capillary blood is obtained by thumb prick and the INR is derived by a biomedical scientist on a small coagulation machine that is dedicated for this purpose. The scientist writes the INR result in the Yellow Book.

- **Option 1:** If the INR is **within** range (e.g. 2.2 in the range 2–3) the patient is verbally recommended to continue taking the same daily dose. The Yellow Book is retained and the patient is told they will receive it in the post, and then sent home. The Yellow Book is then passed to a second room where the dosing officer (perhaps a scientist or pharmacist) will write in their recommendation and enter the details on a computer. The computer then offers a future appointment (up to a maximum of 12 weeks) that the DO writes in the Yellow Book. At the end of the clinic all retained Yellow Books are posted out 1st class to the patients by a clerical assistant.

- **Option 2:** If the INR is out of range (e.g. 1.3 or 3.6 in the range 2–3) the patient (taking their Yellow Book with them) is invited to consult in the adjoining room with the DO to discuss the abnormal result. The DO invites suggestions for causes (e.g. missed doses, use of antibiotics, change of dose of another drug). The DO then decides/negotiates appropriate action (i.e. increase/decrease daily dose) and, with the help of the computer, offers the patient a future appointment to re-test their INR. The patient then leaves, taking their Yellow Book with them.

Training

The NPSA safety alert emphasises that all staff interacting with anticoagulant control of patients will be appropriately trained. This is likely to be organised by the Thrombosis Committee and delivered by a senior scientist.

Other models

In another model patients are venesected from an ante-cubital vein in Out-patients, or in a side room of the laboratory. The patients then wait as their blood passes (via porter or pneumatic chute) to the laboratory for INR generation which is telephoned back to clinic. The DO then consults directly with the patient and notes are made in the Yellow Book. Patients may be offered a targeted appointment (e.g. 10.15 am) or are invited to attend at any time within the three hours of a session. This model therefore saves some effort in out-patient clinics but places more stress on the phlebotomy service and the main laboratory.

Beyond the hospital

The safety and efficacy of oral anticoagulant therapy (essentially, warfarin) is such that it can be transferred from the hospital to general practice. Several models exist:

A: Patients are venesected at their practice, generally by the practice nurse, who retains the Yellow Book. The blood tube passes to the local DGH laboratory (van, post) where the INR is generated. Results are passed back to the GP (telephone, fax, email) for them to manage to patient (via the Yellow Book) as appropriate.

B: As above, but the Yellow Book is also passed to the hospital where the INR is generated. The DO later contacts the patient directly (at home/mobile) with recommendations to remain on the same dose or change to a different daily dose as appropriate, and return as necessary. The Yellow Book is returned to the patient by post.

C: The local DGH provides the scientific personnel and equipment for the practice to generate an INR immediately from the patient, probably by thumb prick. The results and Yellow Book are then taken back to the hospital for computer-assisted dosing, and patients are then managed from the hospital as (B) above.

D: As C, but patient's result is immediately translated into a recommendation by a local DO provided by the hospital who is equipped with a laptop computer loaded with the dosing software. The DO then consults immediately with the patients. This then is essentially an entire hospital out-patient clinic transferred to the practice.

E: The practice runs their own clinic with a near-patient-testing (NPT) device completely independent of the hospital.

Naturally each model has associated logistical and economic implications for the hospital finance officers and the practice managers to consider.

Consolidation (see pages 82–85 for answers)

7.5 What is the general method for changing a patient's warfarin dose to ensure their INR is in range?

7.6 What is the approximate average daily dose of warfarin taken by low-risk patients?

7.7 What is the approximate average daily dose of warfarin taken by high-risk patients?

7.8 What patient factors influence the dose of warfarin?

Case Study 4

In the 24th September warfarin clinic, an 80-year-old woman with a long-standing artificial mechanical heart valve and a history of cardiovascular disease is sent in to see the dosing officer with her Yellow Book. It has the following history:

Date	INR	Recommended daily dose	Next visit (weeks)
4th May	3.8	3mg/4mg alternate days	3
25th May	3.2	Same dose	4
22nd June	3.9	Same dose	3
13th August	4.1	Same dose	3
3rd September	3.8	Same dose	4
24th September	4.3		

What are your questions and what is your recommendation?

N.b. In one clinical trial of people with a form of artificial heart valve, patients randomised to dabigatran fared worse than those randomised to warfarin. Therefore in this case, a NOAC is not necessarily the preferred anticoagulant.

Chapter 8

Use of NOACs

Although powerful therapeutics, the disadvantages of the traditional anticoagulants (heparins, VKAs) (Table 8.1) prompted the development of better agents.

Figure 1.1 shows a rough outline of the process of clot (thrombus) formation, whilst Figure 8.1 summarises key aspects of the coagulation pathway, with emphasis on the parts played by Factor Xa and thrombin.

Because of their key position, these two molecules are ideal candidates for drugs to inhibit thrombosis. These drugs are therefore called direct Factor Xa inhibitors and direct thrombin inhibitors respectively, and in recognising that they work in a different manner to warfarin, are collectively called non-vitamin K antagonist oral anticoagulants (NOACs). They may also be referred to as Direct Oral Anticoagulants.

Table 8.1 Disadvantages of traditional anticoagulants

Vitamin K antagonists	<ul><li>Regular blood tests (perhaps 4-weekly, hence expensive and inconvenient to manage)</li><li>Narrow therapeutic window</li><li>Interactions with many other drugs</li><li>Teratogenic</li><li>Long-half life (hence insensitive to need for a rapid change)</li></ul>
Unfractionated heparin	<ul><li>Need to be injected</li><li>Requirement for monitoring with activated partial thromboplastin time</li><li>Small risk of heparin-induced thrombocytopenia</li></ul>
Low molecular weight heparin	<ul><li>Need to be injected</li><li>Very small risk of heparin-induced thrombocytopenia</li></ul>

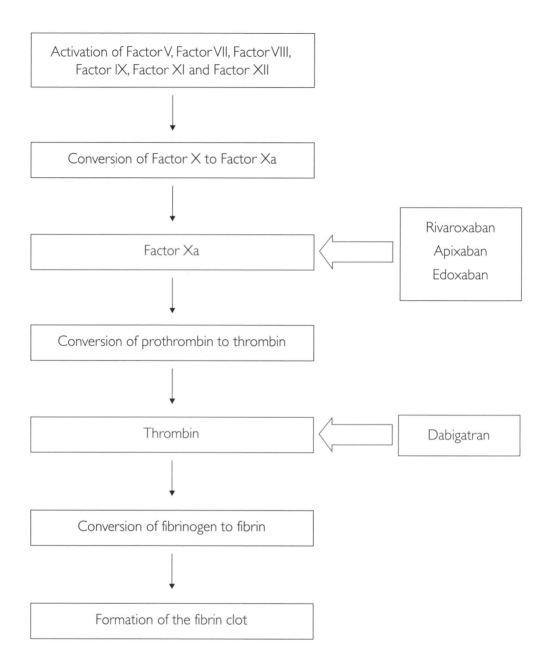

Figure 8.1

**Key aspects of the coagulation pathway
showing the action of NOACs**

At present, there is only one direct thrombin inhibitor on the market (dabigatran), but several Factor Xa inhibitors (rivaroxaban, apixaban, edoxaban). Recognising the mode of action, they all carry the suffix –xaban. This is reminiscent of other classes of drugs, such as the ACE inhibitors (-pril: ramapril) and beta-blockers (-lol: bisoprolol). These drugs were brought to market after the establishment of NICE, and therefore have been subjected to rigorous evaluation in the form of a 'technology appraisal' (TA). Those drugs in the act of being assessed are given the notation of 'In development' (ID), and a full TA will eventually be published. Table 8.2 shows the TA and ID numbers for the indication of each NOAC.

Table 8.2 NICE documents and the NOACs

Indication	NOAC	NICE document
VTE following hip and knee orthopaedic surgery	Dabigatran	TA157
	Rivaroxaban	TA170
	Apixaban	TA245
Stroke and systemic embolism in AF	Dabigatran	TA249
	Rivaroxaban	TA256
	Apixaban	TA275
	Edoxaban	ID624
Prevention and treatment of VTE after acute DVT	Dabigatran	ID483
	Rivaroxaban	TA261
	Apixaban	ID726
	Edoxaban	ID622

VTE: venous thromboembolism. DVT: deep vein thrombosis. TA: technology appraisal.
ID: in development. See www.NICE.org.uk

Like all drugs, we must consider renal function and co-medications – that is, cautions and contra-indications. Details of these for each of the NOACs are presented in Tables 8.3 and 8.4. Regarding renal failure, the dose of the NOACs must be reduced to avoid overdose and so haemorrhage, and in some cases a NOAC is contra-indicated. The same principles (NOAC dose reduction, contra-indication) apply to certain co-medications. If the patient is due to be admitted to hospital for surgery, the NOAC dose (like that of warfarin) will need to be reduced or stopped for a period of time, as summarised in Table 8.5.

Table 8.3 Renal function and the NOACs

	Dabigatran	Apixaban	Rivaroxaban
Fraction of absorbed dose that is renally excreted	80%	27%	35%
Half-life when CrCl ≥60ml/min	~14 hours	No data	~8.5 hours
Half-life when CrCl 30–60ml/min	~18 hours	No data	~9 hours
Half-life when CrCl 15–30ml/min	~28 hours	No data	~9.5 hours
Not recommended if CrCl ≤	30ml/min	15ml/min	15ml/min
Dosing recommendation when creatinine clearance is falling	CrCl 30–49ml/min: reduce dose, e.g. from 150 to 110mg bd	CrCl 15–29ml/min: reduce dose, e.g. from 5 to 2.5mg bd	CrCl 15–49ml/min: reduce dose, e.g. from 20 to 10mg qd

CrCl – creatinine clearance

Table 8.4 Selected drug interactions with NOACs

Drug	Dabigatran	Apixaban	Rivaroxaban
Atorvastatin	+18%	No data yet	No effect
Verapamil	+12–80%***	No data yet	Minor effect*
Quinidine	+50%***	No data yet	+50%***
Diltiazem	No effect	+40%***	Minor effect*
Amiodarone	+12–60%***	No data yet	Minor effect*
Dronadarone	+70–100%**	No data yet	No data yet
Ketoconazole, itraconazole, voriconazole, posaconazole	+140–150%**	+100%**	Up to +160%**
Clarithromycin, erythromycin	+15–20%***	No data yet	+30–54%***
Rifampicin, St John's Wort, carbamazepine, phenytoin, phenobarbital	-66%**	-54%**	Up to -50%
Antacids (e.g. H2 blockers, proton pump inhibitors)	-12–30%	No data yet	No effect

*Use with caution if creatinine clearance 15–50ml/min. **Use contra-indicated/not recommended. ***Reduce the dose of the NOAC. N.b. this list is not intended to be exhaustive.

Table 8.5 Last intake of drug before elective surgical intervention

	Dabigatran		Apixaban		Rivaroxaban	
	Low risk – high risk		Low risk – high risk		Low risk – high risk	
CrCl ≥80ml/min	≥24	≥48	≥24	≥48	≥24	≥48
CrCl 50–80ml/min	≥36	≥72	≥24	≥48	≥24	≥48
CrCl 30–50ml/min*	≥48	≥96	≥24	≥48	≥24	≥48
CrCl 15–30ml/min*	Not indicated		≥36	≥48	≥36	≥48

Use of any NOAC is not indicated when creatinine clearance (CrCl) is <15ml/min. Data is time in hours before surgery when treatment is to be stopped. *Many patients may be on the lower doses of the NOAC.

The NOACs

Dabigatran

The first NOAC to market, dabigatran possesses various qualities which make it potentially an attractive and promising OAC with its predictable pharmacokinetics and pharmacodynamics. The drug has rapid absorption (within 2 hours) and distribution with estimated half-lives of 8–10 hours and 14–17 hours for single and multiple dose administrations, respectively. Nearly 80% is excreted unchanged by the kidneys with average bioavailability of 6.5%, hence high doses are required to maintain adequate plasma concentrations. Of note, the drug absorption is reduced by 20–25% if patients are concurrently on proton pump inhibitors. Although clinical trials have been conducted assessing dosages, efficacy and tolerability in numerous indications such as prevention of secondary VTE, DVT, stroke and embolism due to AF, it is licensed only for the prevention of VTE following orthopaedic surgery and in atrial fibrillation (Table 8.2).

Rivaroxaban

This drug is the first selective oral direct Factor Xa inhibitor advanced to clinical trials. With favourable pharmacokinetic characteristics and a bioavailability of 60–80%, rivaroxaban achieves peak plasma levels in 3 hours and has a half-life of 9 hours in healthy, young subjects and about 12 hours in elderly subjects – however, the drug has been tested for clinical use on once daily basis. It is metabolised by the liver with up to two-thirds of the drug being eliminated by the kidneys. Caution in the use of rivaroxaban in patients with renal impairment is required because of its renal clearance. It does not significantly interact with platelet function in preclinical studies, where it demonstrated an excellent correlation between its plasma levels and achieved clotting times, while the bleeding risk was comparable to that of enoxaparin. Rivaroxaban has also been trialled for the prevention of secondary VTE, DVT, stroke and embolism due to AF, and is licensed for all these indications (Table 8.2).

Apixaban

This highly selective and potent low molecular weight inhibitor of Factor Xa has a bioavailability of more than 50% and half-life of between 9 and 14 hours. Apixaban has fixed twice-daily dosing and is metabolised in the liver, with about 25% excreted by the kidneys and the remainder by intestinal excretion. It has been shown to be safe and well tolerated in initial testing in volunteers and its anticoagulant effects are closely correlated to plasma concentration of the drug. Apixaban too has been trialled for the prevention of secondary VTE, DVT, stroke and embolism due to AF, but like dabigatran is licensed only to prevent VTE after orthopaedic surgery and in AF (Table 8.2).

Edoxaban

This low molecular weight Factor Xa inhibitor, like others in its class, also shows promise in terms of efficacy and safety compared to VKAs. It has a bioavailability of 66%, plasma levels peak 1–2 hours after ingestion, minimal hepatic metabolism, and 50% is excreted via the kidney. It has been trialled in the prevention of secondary VTE, DVT, stroke and embolism due to AF, but as yet is unlicensed in the UK (Table 8.2).

It may be predicted that all NOACs will eventually be licensed by NICE for all indications, i.e. prevention of VTE after orthopaedic surgery, prevention of VTE in AF, and the treatment and prevention of VTE after acute VTE.

NICE documents

NICE CG92. Venous thromboembolism: reducing the risk

This CG offers general advice on the management of VTE, but also on the use of dabigatran and rivaroxaban as alternatives to warfarin and LMWH in the immediate and follow-up stages of elective hip or knee replacement. Provided there are no contra-indications, pharmacological VTE prophylaxis should be started after surgery. The options are:

(a) dabigatran, starting 1–4 hours after surgery,

(b) fondaparinux sodium, starting 6 hours after surgical closure provided haemostasis has been established,

(c) LMWH, starting 6–12 hours after surgery,

(d) rivaroxaban, starting 6–10 hours after surgery, and

(e) UFH (for patients with renal failure), starting 6–12 hours after surgery.

Pharmacological VTE prophylaxis should be continued for 28–35 days after hip replacement, but for 10–14 days after knee replacement. NOACs are not recommended after hip fracture or other orthopaedic surgery. Notably, apixaban is recommended for the prevention of VTE in these situations (TA245) so may be expected to be included in re-writes of CG92.

Frustratingly, the CG does not offer advice on the dose of the NOAC, but this is available in the summary of product characteristics, the particular TA document, and in the BNF (see Table 8.6).

NICE TA261: Rivaroxaban for the treatment of DVT and prevention of recurrent DVT and PE

The traditional treatment of acute symptomatic VTE was a LMWH and warfarin, the LMWH to be stopped once the warfarin was effective (i.e. INR 2–3), generally for 6 months. Clinical trials compared this regime with rivaroxaban, and NICE subsequently recommended a dose of 15mg of rivaroxaban twice a day for three weeks, then 20mg once a day. The guideline also found the NOAC to be more cost-effective than the traditional regime for up to 12 months, and also for a longer period for those in whom extended OAC was required.

NICE TA287: Rivaroxaban for treating PE and preventing recurrent VTE

This appraisal is very similar to TA261 (for those presenting with a DVT), but TA287 instead refers to patients presenting with an acute PE. The recommended dosage is the same, i.e. 15mg twice a day for three weeks, then 20mg once a day (15mg in moderate or severe renal failure) for continued treatment.

NICE CG180: Atrial fibrillation: the management of atrial fibrillation

Atrial fibrillation (AF) is a leading risk factor for stroke. However, not every patient is at the same risk of stroke or systemic embolism. This risk varies from individual to individual according to a number of clinical and demographic factors that include chronic heart failure, hypertension, age, diabetes mellitus, previous stroke or transient ischaemic attack, female sex, and other cardiovascular disease (such as myocardial infarction). Together, these give a mathematical risk of a major event that an individual AF patient carries, and this overall risk has been fashioned into the clinical scoring systems of CHA_2DS_2VASc. Each risk factor carries a score of 1, but stroke or transient ischaemic attack carries a score of 2, age 65–74 scores 1 whilst age 75 or greater scores 2. The higher the score, the greater the risk of thrombosis and so the greater the need for anticoagulation.

However, anticoagulation also brings a risk of haemorrhage, and the likelihood of this can be assessed by the HAS-BLED score, a sum of hypertension, abnormal renal/liver function, stroke, bleeding history or predisposition, labile International Normalised Ratio, elderly and drugs/alcohol concomitantly. Each factor scores 1, and the higher the HAS-BLED score, the greater the risk of haemorrhage. By comparing the risk of haemorrhage (as HAS-BLED) with the protection from stroke (as CHA_2DS_2VASc) an overall view of the net clinical benefit of anticoagulation can be obtained. However, HAS-BLED is neither designed nor validated as a method of denying anticoagulation; instead it draws attention to those patients who may require more care.

NICE CG180 recommends that both CHA_2DS_2VASc and HAS-BLED be used to determine suitability for anticoagulation. It also refers to options of any of the three NOACs or a VKA. In order to help practitioners decide, a third scoring system has been developed, based on the likelihood of achieving a good time in therapeutic range (TTR), that is, an INR between 2 and 3 for at least

70% of the time, when taking a VKA. In this model female sex (marked by S), age (A) less than 60 years, medical (Me) history of chronic disease (hypertension, diabetes, cardiovascular disease, or pulmonary, hepatic or renal disease), treatment (T) with certain drugs (such as amiodarone), use of tobacco (T) within the last two years, and non-Caucasian race (R) are all risk factors for a poor TTR. Putting these factors together generates the SAMe-TT$_2$R$_2$ score, where T (tobacco use) and R (non-Caucasian race) both score 2 points, all other factors scoring 1. Thus an individual's likelihood of TTR can be quantified, and if their SAMe-TT$_2$R$_2$ score is 0 or 1, then a VKA (almost inevitably warfarin) is recommended. For those with SAMe-TT$_2$R$_2$ score ≥2, a NOAC is recommended. This is important as those with a poor TTR are at risk of both thrombosis (when the INR is below the target range) and haemorrhage (when above the target range). Regardless of the nature of the AF, once prescribed, anticoagulation is generally for life. Table 8.6 summarises the factors that make up these three scoring systems, whilst Figure 8.2 shows a flow chart for their use in a practical setting.

Table 8.6 Scoring systems for VTE management in AF

CHA$_2$DS$_2$VASc Factor	Score	HAS-BLED Factor	Score	SAMe-TT$_2$R$_2$ Factor	Score
Chronic heart failure	1	Hypertension	1	Sex = Female	1
Hypertension	1	Abnormal liver or renal function	1	Age less than 60	1
Age 65–74	1	Stroke	1	Medical history of chronic disease	1
Age 75 or more	2	Bleeding history	1	Treatment with certain drugs	1
Diabetes	1	Labile INR	1	Tobacco	2
Stroke/TIA	2	Elderly	1	Race: non-Caucasian	2
Vascular disease (e.g. myocardial infarction)	1	Drugs/alcohol	1		
Sex category (female)	1				
Maximum score	9	Maximum score	6	Maximum score	8

TIA = transient ischaemic attack, INR = international normalised ratio

The flow chart in Figure 8.2 provides a firm basis for decision making; the upper part is approved by NICE and the European Cardiology Society. However, the final part of the process is missing: the choice of a particular NOAC. This is difficult because each has its own advantages and disadvantages. Some suggest that rivaroxaban is preferable as it is a once-a-day prescription; others prefer apixaban as it has a lower risk of haemorrhage. Accordingly, the practitioner should consider the options alongside the patient. Table 8.7 summarises the indications and doses of the NOACs.

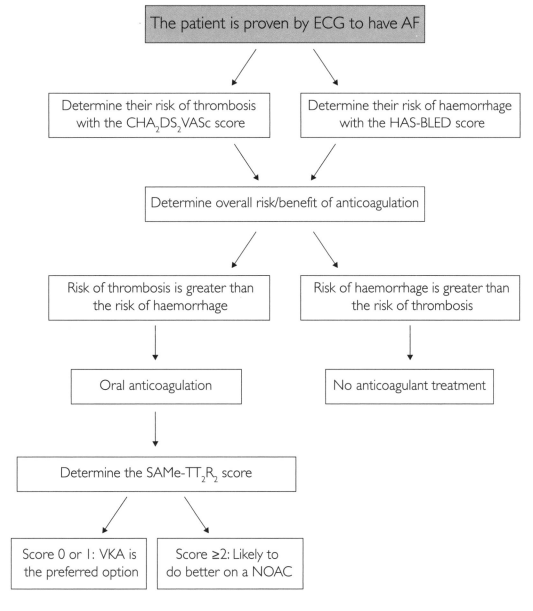

Figure 8.2
Management of the risk of VTE in AF

Table 8.7 Doses of NOACs for defined indications

NOAC	Indication	Dose
Dabigatran	Orthopaedic surgery (TA157)	An initial dose of 110mg, then 220mg od. However, the initial dose may be 75mg and the following doses 110mg in those with moderate CKD, the elderly, and those on amiodarone
	Atrial fibrillation (TA249)	150mg bd, reduced to 110mg od at physician's discretion at ages 75–80, but to 75mg for all aged 80 or over
Apixaban	Orthopaedic surgery (TA245)	2.5mg bd
	Atrial fibrillation (TA275)	5mg bd, but 2.5mg in those at a high risk of haemorrhage (e.g. the elderly)
Rivaroxaban	Orthopaedic surgery (TA170)	10mg od
	Atrial fibrillation (TA256)	20mg od (15mg in those at high risk of haemorrhage)
	Acute DVT or PE (TA261, TA287)	15mg bd for 21 days, then 20mg od

TA = technology appraisal, CKD = chronic kidney disease, od = once daily, bd = twice daily

Consolidation (see pages 82–85 for answers)

8.1 Why are NOACs preferred to traditional agents in certain indications?

8.2 What medical factors must be considered in the use of NOACs?

8.3 What is the difference between a NICE clinical guideline and a technology appraisal?

8.4 Which of the NOACs can be used to prevent VTEs after orthopaedic surgery?

8.5 People with AF are not at a very high risk of VTE, so why do they need to be anticoagulated?

Case Study 5

An 84-year-old obese (body mass index 31.5kg/m^2) Afro-Caribbean man with a history of peripheral vascular disease (reduced ankle-brachial pressure index) is diagnosed with AF. He has benign prostatic hyperplasia and is taking finasteride. He is also taking aspirin 75mg od and amlodipine 5mg od, his blood pressure being found to be 144/92 and he does not smoke.

How do you determine whether or not he should be anticoagulated, and if so, with what?

Chapter 9

What happens if something goes wrong? – Haemorrhage

What is haemorrhage?

The consequences of over-anticoagulation can be many and varied, Examples of haemorrhage include bloodshot eyes, blood in mouth after brushing teeth, bleeding after shaving, bruising over arms/legs etc. How seriously should this be taken? Certainly, vomiting and urinating blood are serious and demand attention. But how much blood has been lost? An obvious answer is to look for a reduction in the haemoglobin level of the full blood count. Generally, a 20-unit fall is considered serious and may demand a blood transfusion. This, of course, demands a recent FBC. Degrees of haemorrhage are summarised in Table 9.1, the most serious probably being a haemorrhagic stroke.

Table 9.1 Degrees of haemorrhage

Level	Typical clinical picture
1	Relatively minor and localised bruising, especially at sites of trauma
2a	Extensive bruising caused by trauma.
2b	Extensive spontaneous bruising in the (claimed/presumed) absence of trauma
3	Actual bleeding, such as epistaxis, and bleeding from gums and wounds
4	Haematuria, vomiting blood, bleeding per vagina, per rectum
5	Major bleeding: from or into a critical organ, such as intra-cranial, intra-spinal, gastro-intestinal, intra-ocular, retroperitoneal, intra-articular, pericardial or intramuscular, and/or a fall in Hb >20 g/L, leading to the transfusion of two or more units of whole blood or red cells.

In the face of clear haemorrhage, the initial response is to stop the next dose of the drug, then consider options, which are likely to include a blood test. The drug may need to be stopped for several days, and if there is a great loss of blood, or if it is likely, then more active treatment with fluids and blood components (prothrombin complex concentrate, etc.) is needed.

IMPORTANT

This scheme is based on practice but is **NOT** to be taken as useable in your setting.

Your local anticoagulant service will have their own scheme written by the Thrombosis Committee and based on firm national and/or international guidelines.

Heparin

Because unfractionated heparin and LMWHs have a short half-life, problems can often resolve quite rapidly by simply stopping the treatment. However, serious haemorrhage (definition – as for warfarin) is treated by protamine sulphate (non-proprietary or Prosul; see the BNF) given by slow IV infusion. Generally, 1mg neutralises 80–100 units of heparin. The maximum dose is 50mg as an excess can have an anticoagulant effect. Curiously, cautions for the use of protamine sulphate include fish allergy, men who are infertile or who have had a vasectomy. However, the problems are almost always ward-based and due to unfractionated heparin.

The degree of anticoagulation of the blood can be determined by the APTT or by the anti-Factor Xa blood tests for unfractionated heparin and LMWH respectively.

Warfarin

An increasing INR brings a risk of haemorrhage that demands action as it may be fatal or at least seriously debilitating (e.g. haemorrhagic stroke). A major problem is that as warfarin has a long half-life, changes are slow and so will not be evident in less than a few days.

In the case of an effective overdose of warfarin, options are to reduce or stop the drug and give the antidote, vitamin K. Responses depend on whether or not the patient is an in-patient or an out-patient.

High INR in an out-patient

Therapeutic decisions are dependent on the INR, whether or not there is minor or major bleeding, other risk factors for bleeding (e.g. age >70 years, previous bleeding complications), and the reason for anticoagulation (AF/post VTE/post-surgical?). See Table 9.2.

Table 9.2 Action in response to a high INR in an out-patient

INR	Action
3.1–3.5 (only if target INR 2.5)	Consider same dose (e.g. if 3.1) or reduce by about 5% (e.g. if 3.5). Re-test in 2–5 days
3.6–3.9 (only if target INR 2.5)	Reduce dose by about 5–10%. Re-test in 1–5 days
4.0–5.9	Consider stopping warfarin for 1–2 days. Recommence warfarin on reduced dose (about 10–15%). Re-test within 2–5 days
6.0–6.9	Stop warfarin for 2–3 days. Recommence warfarin on reduced dose (about 15–20%). Re-test in 1–4 days
7.0–7.9	Stop warfarin for 2–3 days. Recommence warfarin on reduced dose (about 20–30%). Re-test next day
8.0–8.9	Stop warfarin. Consider vitamin K oral 1.0mg. Re-test next day
9.0–11.9	Stop warfarin. Consider vitamin K oral 1.0–2.0mg, re-test next day
12.0–14.9	Inform Consultant Haematologist. Give vitamin K, oral, 2mg. Stop warfarin. Re-test next day.
15.0–20.0	Inform Consultant Haematologist. Give vitamin K oral 2.5–5.0mg. Stop warfarin. Re-test the next day

In all cases the patient's current warfarin dose stability, concurrent medications and clinical condition must be considered when advising dose change and date of re-test. One or two days of a reduced dose may be worthwhile in some cases before resumption of the new dose. Significant bleeding (e.g. haematuria) with any INR result should be discussed with a haematologist. Anticoagulant services will refer those patients with marked haemorrhage to A&E immediately, and will inform A&E of their imminent arrival.

Any out-patient receiving OACs who may be experiencing a major bleeding episode should be advised to seek urgent medical attention from the nearest A&E department.

High INR in an in-patient

Clearly, being an in-patient implies some serious medical or surgical issue. 'Need to knows' include INR, any current or previous bleeding, reason for anticoagulation, patient age/diagnosis (elderly patients are more likely to bleed, but generally need less warfarin). Bleeding at therapeutic INR needs investigation for local cause.

Other diagnoses, e.g. cardiac failure (hence need to know left ventricle ejection fraction), liver dysfunction (hence need to request LFTs), renal dysfunction (hence need to request urea, creatinine and electrolytes) are relevant not only in identifying the cause but also in predicting responses to treatment. Action is directed by Table 9.3.

Table 9.3 Action in response to a high INR in an in-patient

INR	Action
3.1–6.0 (only if target INR 2.5)	Reduce warfarin dose or stop. Re-start when INR<5.0
4.0–6.0 (only if target INR 3.5)	Reduce warfarin dose or stop. Re-start when INR<5.0
6.0–8.0 No bleeding or minor bleeding	Stop warfarin. Re-start when INR <5.0, consider vitamin K 0.5–1.0mg orally
>8.0 No bleeding or minor bleeding	Stop warfarin. Re-start when INR<5.0 if wish to anticoagulate again. If other risk factors for bleeding, give 2.5mg vitamin K oral or IV (for INRs 12–20 give 5mg vitamin K). Repeat dose of vitamin K after 24 hrs if INR still high. Seek advice
Major bleeding	Stop warfarin. Give prothrombin complex concentrate (Beriplex) 50 units/kg or FFP 15ml/kg. Give 5mg vitamin K IV. Repeat dose of vitamin K after 24 hrs if INR still high. Seek advice

Intravenous vitamin K rarely causes allergy and is safe. The IV preparation 'Konakion MM Paediatric' can be given orally. The degree of reversal with vitamin K varies on an individual basis, e.g. patients with prosthetic valves may require blood components only and a very small dose of vitamin K to avoid oral anticoagulant resistance later. IV vitamin K reverses more rapidly than oral vitamin K and should be used if reversal is urgent.

NOACs

As with warfarin, step one is to stop the next dose of the drug, and then determine, as accurately as possible, the time of the last dose of the drug. With a short half-life, action in view of actual or potential haemorrhage has similarities with that of unfractionated and LMWH. However, there are as yet no antidotes, although several are well into the development process.

Action may call for knowledge of the degree of anticoagulation of the patient's blood. This will be a blood test, dependent on the NOAC itself. The local laboratory will know what to do, and will ask for a 'coagulation' vacutainer: light blue top with sodium citrate (as for an INR). As with other drugs, there may in theory be a need for fluids and blood components, and re-starting must then be considered.

Practical response to a haemorrhage

If bleeding is serious, then action is needed to maintain haemodynamics (blood volume), possibly to maintain the red cell count and haemoglobin (rarely needed, but if so, blood transfusion), and to correct the abnormal coagulation system and so maintain haemostasis. All of these will be done in secondary care, so that severe bleeding in primary care demands a 999 call. If there is bleeding from a wound, this may be compressed and/or bound tightly. Active direct intervention possibilities are as follows:

- Maintain diuresis (drinking water)
- Saline: provides only haemodynamic support in restoring lost blood volume
- Consider tranexamic acid and desmopressin (to stimulate the endothelium to secrete pro-coagulants)
- Packed red cells: to restore lost oxygen-carrying capacity
- Platelet concentrates: to correct a thrombocytopenia
- Fresh frozen plasma: to help correct plasma volume (not to correct haemostasis)
- Activated Factor VII (Factor VIIa)
- Prothrombin complex concentrate (PCC), such as Beriplex
- Activated PCC (Feiba, actually developed for use in haemophilia)
- For Xa-inhibitors, consider PCC (25 units/kg: may be repeated once or twice), activated PCC (e.g., Feiba, 40–80 units/kg, maximum 200 units/kg/day), recombinant Factor VIIa, (e.g. 90 µg/kg).
- For dabigatran, as for Xa-inhibitors, but also consider concentrates of coagulation Factors II, IX and X. Consider charcoal and dialysis.

After an appropriate period, determine likelihood of the return of haemostasis with drug-specific blood tests.

Causes of haemorrhage

An attempt must be made to establish the cause of over-anticoagulation in case this impacts upon further treatment. Consideration should be given to the need for the patient to continue on anticoagulation in the presence of contra-indications, e.g. age, non-compliance. But without doubt the leading cause of haemorrhage is drug interaction, and of these, antibiotics are the main culprits.

Other established risk factors include patient confusion, recent return from holiday, age, binge use of alcohol, and inadequate education leading to poor compliance (especially warfarin). Significant drug interactions are listed in appendix I of the BNF and identified with a black spot. If the patient has bled as a result of the interaction or requires admission to hospital a yellow card should be completed and sent to The Medicines and Healthcare Products Regulatory Agency (MHRA).

As regards warfarin, the interactions section of the BNF has 30 bullet points on drugs that may interfere with the activity of warfarin. Some are listed in Table 9.4. Interactions of NOACs with other medications are outlined in Table 8.4 (p. 62).

Table 9.4 Some drug interactions with warfarin

Analgesics:	NSAIDS, celecoxib, ibuprofen, diclofenac, aspirin, paracetamol
Antibacterials:	Neomycin, chloroamphenicol, erythromycin
Antidepressants:	Venlafaxine, St John's Wort, tricyclics
Cytotoxics:	Fluorouracil, azathioprine, mercaptopurine
Lipid-regulators	Colestryramine, rosuvastatin, fibrates, simvastatin
Ulcer-healers	Cimitidine, esomeprazole, omeprazole, sulcralfate

Curiously, cranberry juice seems likely to interact with warfarin. But if a drug interaction is suspected and/or can be predicted, it may be necessary to alter the dose of the particular drug and/or that of warfarin. But which way? And which drug is more important? Increased monitoring is likely.

Patient reassurance and education

It is likely that the haemorrhaging patient (whether on warfarin, NOAC or heparin) will be very concerned and so reassurance is required. In addition, this will provide an opportunity to reinforce patient education with regards to risk factors and concomitant medications.

Consolidation (see pages 82–85 for answers)

9.1 What is the antidote for excess heparin?

9.2 What are the first actions in cases of excess warfarin or a NOAC?

9.3 What are the treatments for life-threatening haemorrhage?

9.4 Which commonly prescribed drugs interact with warfarin?

Case Study 6

A 65-year-old man with no English visits the anticoagulation clinic with his wife and an interpreter. The indication for warfarin is DVT and his duration of treatment is 6 months. His Yellow Book gives the following history, starting with 6mg, but 7mg on Wednesdays and Sundays.

Date (weeks)	INR	Recommended daily dose	Next visit
8th October	2.5	Same dose	3
22nd October	1.5	Same dose	1
29th October	2.9	Same dose	2
12th November	4.0	Miss one dose, then resume	1
19th November	3.1	Same dose	2
3rd December	1.2	6mg/7mg alternate days	1
10th December	2.8	Same dose	2
24th December	8.5	Stop warfarin, 1mg vitamin K given	(4 days)
28th December	3.2	5mg daily	(3 days)
31st December	2.1	6mg daily	1
7th January	1.5	6mg/7mg alternate days	1
14th January	1.3	7mg daily	1
21st January	3.6		

What to do?

Case Study 7

A 56-year-old man comes in to see you in the oral anticoagulant clinic in extreme anxiety because the sclera (the white part) of his left eye is completely red. You admit it looks bad. He says that he had an irritation in the eye a few days ago and rubbed it hard for several minutes. His INR is 2.4 (target 2.5).

What to do?

Case Study 8

A 63-year-old woman comes to the oral anticoagulant clinic in advance of her appointment. She reports a history of occasional blood in her urine over the past ten days, and has had two nosebleeds. Her INR today is 8.5.

What to do?

Case Study 9

A 77-year-old Afro-Caribbean woman with AF has recently been transferred from warfarin to rivaroxaban. She reported blood on the toilet paper after defaecation, and a subsequent faecal occult blood test was positive. An investigation with a colonoscopy found evidence of intestinal mucosal haemorrhage. What are the options for future OAC?

Summary

VTE is far from a benign condition: ten years after thrombosis:
- Over half of patients (56%) will have suffered post-thrombotic syndrome
- 29% will have suffered a recurrent VTE
- 28% will be dead: mostly from cancer, myocardial infarction or stroke.

VTEs, comprising DVT and PE, are common and treatable both in hospital and in the community. Established treatments are as follows:

- **Warfarin** is a most effective oral anticoagulant. However, misuse confers a significant risk of bleeding, there is no common dose, it is difficult to control, and is sensitive to numerous commonly prescribed drugs. Yet, despite these drawbacks, it remains a powerful agent for the reduction of various VTEs in many different circumstances.
- Developed from unfractionated heparin, **LMWH** is a choice in many conditions where thrombosis is to be avoided or, at least, minimised. However, recent guidelines for the use of unfractionated heparin suggest some value.

- **NOACs** are slowly becoming established and appearing in guidelines for specific indications such as after orthopaedic surgery and in AF. They do not need routine blood test monitoring and are safer than warfarin.

Treatment agent(s) and duration (3 months, 6 months, life) depend on the persistence of the cause/ risk factor. Major risk factors include increasing age, recent surgery (especially orthopaedic), cancer (especially active) and thrombophilia.

Tips for practitioners

When faced with a patient with suspected or actual DVT or PE, relevant steps (often in collaboration with secondary care) include:

- Assess the clinical state of the patient, e.g. symptoms, haemodynamic stability, etc.
- Assess risk factors for a DVT or PE, and manage the correctable ones.
- Assess the diagnostic probability of a DVT or PE.
- If DVT, consider out-patient management or referral to specialist centre. If PE suspected, refer to hospital.
- Have a clear management plan with regard to treatment (warfarin and/or LMWH, NOAC) and the duration of such treatment, often in consultation with hospital. The management plan will inevitably refer to recent authoritative guidelines.
- In view of the risk of recurrence, consider prophylactic measures (e.g. GECS, etc.) where appropriate (degree of risk, immobility, pre-surgery, etc.).

Selected references

General and Epidemiology

Anderson, F.A. & Spencer, F.A. (2003). Risk factors for venous thromboembolism. *Circulation* **107**: I-9 – I-16.

Anderson, F.A. & Wheeler, H.B. (1992). Physician practices in the management of VTE. *Journal of Vascular Surgery* **16**: 707–14.

Anonymous (2006). Treat DVT out of hospital with subcutaneous heparin. *British Medical Journal* **333**: 543.

Bates, S.M., Greer, I.A., Hirsh, J. et al. (2004). Use of antithrombotic agents during pregnancy. *Chest* **126** (Suppl 3): 627S-44S.

Bauer, K.A. (2013). Pros and cons of new oral anticoagulants. Hematology: *American Society of Hematology Education Program.* 2013: 464–70.

Blann, A.D. (2013). *Routine Blood Results Explained.* 3rd edn. Keswick: M&K Update.

Blann, A.D. & Lip, G.Y.H. (2006). Venous thromboembolism. *British Medical Journal* **332**: 215–19.

British Committee for Standards in Haematology (2006). Guidelines on use of vena cava filters. *British Journal of Haematolology* **134**: 590–5.

Buller, H.R., Sohne, M. & Middeldorp, S. (2005). Treatment of VTE. *Journal of Thrombosis and Haemostasis* **3**: 1554–60.

Cohen, A., Drost, P., Marchant, N., et al. (2012). The efficacy and safety of pharmacological prophylaxis of venous thromboembolism following elective knee or hip replacement: systematic review and network meta-analysis. *Clinical and Applied Thrombosis/Hemostasis* **18**: 611–27.

Cowell, R.P.W. (2014). Direct oral anticoagulants: integration into clinical practice. *Postgraduate Medical Journal* **90**: 529–39.

Golderhaber, S.Z. & Turpie, A.G.G. (2005). Prevention of VTE among hospitalized medical patients. *Circulation* **111**: e1–e3.

Heit, J.A. (2005). VTE: disease burden, outcomes and risk factors. *Journal of Thrombosis and Haemostasis* **3**: 1611–17.

Kher, A., Bauersachs, R., & Nielsen, J.D. (2007). The management of thrombosis in pregnancy. *Thrombosis and Haemostasis* **97**: 505–13

Ost, D., Tepper, J., Mihara, H. et al. (2005). Duration of anticoagulation following VTE. *Journal of the American Medical Association* **294**: 706–15.

Cancer

Donnellan, E., Kevane, B., Bird, B.R. & Ainle, F.N. (2014). Cancer and venous thromboembolic disease: from molecular mechanisms to clinical management. *Current Oncology* **21**: 134–43.

Farge, D., Debourdeau, P., Beckers, M. et al. (2013). International clinical practice guidelines for the treatment and prophylaxis of venous thromboembolism in patients with cancer. *Journal of Thrombosis and Haemostasis* **11**: 56–70.

Lee, A.Y.Y. (2004). Management of thrombosis in cancer. *British Journal of Haematology* **128**: 291–302.

Lin, J., Wakefield, T.W. & Henke, P.K. (2006). Risk factors associated with VTEs in patients with malignancy. *Blood Coagulation and Fibrinolysis* **17**: 265–70.

Lyman, G.H., Khorana, A.A., Kuderer, N.M. et al. (2013). Venous thromboembolism prophylaxis and treatment in patients with cancer: American Society of Clinical Oncology clinical practice guideline update. *Journal of Clinical Oncology* **31**: 2189–204.

Nierodzik, M. & Karpatkin, S. (2005). Hypercoagulability preceding cancer. *Journal of Thrombosis and Haemostasis* **3**: 577–80.

Shea-Budgell, M.A., Wu, C.M. & Easaw, J.C. (2014). Evidence-based guidance on venous thromboembolism in patients with solid tumours. *Current Oncology* **21**: e504–14.

Diagnosis

Fancher, T.L., White, R.H. & Kravitz, R.L. (2004). Combined use of rapid D-dimer and estimation of clinical probability in the diagnosis of DVT: systematic review. *British Medical Journal* **329**: 821.

Ho, W.H., Hankey, G.J., Lee, C.H. & Eikelboom, J.W. (2005). VTE: Diagnosis and managements of DVT. *Medical Journal of Australia* **182**: 476–81.

Kearon, C., Ginsberg, J.S., Douketis, J. *et al.* (2006). An evaluation of D-dimer in the diagnosis of pulmonary embolism: a randomised trial. *Annals of Internal Medicine* **144**: 812–21.

Lee, C.H., Hankey, G.J., Ho, W.H. & Eikelboom, J.W. (2005). VTE: Diagnosis and management of PE. *Medical Journal of Australia* **182**: 569–74.

Guidelines

Baglin, T.P., Keeling, D.M., Watson, H.G., *et al.* (2005). Guidelines on oral anticoagulation (warfarin). *British Journal of Haematology* **132**: 277–85.

Baglin, T.P., Barrowcliffe, T.W., Cohen, A. & Greaves, M. (2006). Guidelines on the use and monitoring of heparin. *British Journal of Haematology* **133**: 19–34.

Baglin, T.P. *et al.* (2007). Safety indicators for inpatient and outpatient oral anticoagulant care. *British Journal of Haematology* **136**: 26–9.

Camm, A.J., Lip, G.Y., De Caterina, R. *et al.* (2012). 2012 focused update of the ESC Guidelines for the management of atrial fibrillation: an update of the 2010 ESC Guidelines for the management of atrial fibrillation – developed with the special contribution of the European Heart Rhythm Association. *Europace* **14**: 1385–413.

Cushman, M., Lim, W. & Zakai, N.A. (2014). *Clinical Practice Guide on Antithrombotic Drug Dosing and Management of Antithrombotic Drug-associated Bleeding Complications in Adults.* Washington DC: American Society of Hematology. Available at: http://www.hematology.org/Clinicians/Guidelines-Quality/Quick-Ref/2869.aspx (last accessed October 2014).

Hirsch, J., Guyatt, G., Albers, G. *et al.* (2004). Seventh ACCP Conference on anti-thrombotic and thromboembolic therapy. *Chest* **126** (3 Suppl): 172S–696S.

Haemorrhage

Awad, N.I., & Cocchio, C. (2013). Activated prothrombin complex concentrates for the reversal of anticoagulant-associated coagulopathy. *P&T* **38**: 696–701.

Steiner, T., Bohm, M., Dichgans, M. *et al.* (2013). Recommendations for the emergency management of complications associated with the new direct oral anticoagulants (DOACs) apixaban, dabigatran and rivaroxaban. *Clinical Research in Cardiology* **102**: 399–412.

Answers to consolidation notes and case studies

Answers to consolidation notes

1.1 What are the two major constituents of a clot?
Fibrin and platelets

1.2 What are the two major coagulation factors in the blood?
Fibrinogen and prothrombin

1.3 What is the name for the process of clot destruction?
Fibrinolysis

1.4 What product of clot destruction can be measured in the plasma?
D-dimers

2.1 Describe some surgical procedures that carry a strong risk of DVT or PE.
Orthopaedic – e.g. hip and knee replacement

2.2 Which risk factors are generally relevant only to women?
During and post-pregnancy, use of the oral contraceptive pill or hormone replacement therapy

2.3 Why do some risk factors seem to promote thrombosis?
By increasing levels of fibrinogen and making platelets more likely to participate in coagulation

2.4 What genetic condition is the most common cause of thrombophilia?
Factor V Leiden – in its heterozygous form is present in 5% of those of white European descent

3.1 What are the most common clinical signs and symptoms of DVT?
Pain, erythema, tenderness and swelling of the affected limb. Findings on examination include a palpable cord (reflecting a thrombosed vein), warmth, oedema or superficial venous dilatation.

3.2 What other aids are there to help diagnosis?
Venography, ultrasound, D-dimers

3.3 What are the most common signs and symptoms of PE?
Dyspnoea, pleuritic pain, cough, tachypnoea, crepitations, tachycardia

3.4 What other aids are there to help a diagnosis?
D-dimers, VQ scanning

4.1 How does warfarin work?
Warfarin is effectively a liver-focused poison that impedes the synthesis of proteins dependent on vitamin K.

4.2 How do we monitor the effect of warfarin on the blood?
We use the International Normalised Ratio, effectively the ratio of the prothrombin time on warfarin compared to the prothrombin time not on warfarin

4.3 Can you name any disadvantages of heparin?
Thrombocytopenia, osteoporosis, alopecia

4.4 Why are NOACs an advance on traditional drugs?
There are several advantages, but the most obvious are that they don't call for a blood test and have a better safety profile.

4.5 What non-drug treatments are available?
Graduated elastic compression stockings, mobility, hydration

5.1 Which single document provides details about all anticoagulants?
The British National Formulary

5.2 What Trust body within your particular workplace should be consulted about best practice?
The Thrombosis Committee

5.3 What is the basis of the risk factor method for providing treatment?
The presumption that different risk factors are more likely to provoke a VTE than others

5.4 Are there patients who should not be given LMWH?
Yes, cautions and contra-indications (Table 5.3) include severe hepatic or renal impairment, major trauma or surgery to the brain, eye or spinal cord, known uncorrected bleeding disorders, thrombocytopenia and allergy.

5.5 What are the options for the long-term treatment and prevention of VTE?
The only feasible option is oral anticoagulation with warfarin (or another VKA), or with a NOAC.

6.1 What 'medical' patients may be in need of anticoagulation?
Those with central venous lines, malignancy (greater if on chemotherapy), congestive heart or respiratory failure (including pneumonia), HRT, use of oral contraceptives, paralytic stroke, post-partum, previous VTE, thrombophilia, bed rest >3 days, immobility due to sitting (e.g. prolonged car or air travel, wheelchair), increasing age, obesity, pregnancy, and varicose veins (i.e. Table 5.1).

6.2 Which patient group should be given aspirin?
Those for whom warfarin and/or heparins are contra-indicated

6.3 What is the most common time of day to give the patient their LMWH?
6 pm, or thereabouts, purely for the convenience of staff doing the drug round

6.4 What is the role of the anaesthetist in providing anticoagulant cover?
The surgeon and anaesthetist are likely to consult over the use of LMWH in terms of the use of general or local anaesthesia (e.g. in epidurals).

6.5 What are the alternatives to LMWH?

The alternatives to LMWH in orthopaedic surgery are one of the NOACs.

7.1 What government agency has published a major document on the general management of warfarin?

The National Patient Safety Agency (NPSA)

7.2 Why should patients about to undergo surgery be taken off warfarin and what is the alternative anticoagulant?

Almost all patients about to undergo more than 30 minutes surgery are likely to be taken off warfarin and given a LMWH.

7.3 How long should treatment with warfarin last?

For as long as the risk factor outweighs the side effects of warfarin – generally 3 months, 6 months or for life

7.4 What kinds of patients require rapid induction or slow induction of warfarin?

This depends on how acute is/are the risk factor(s) for VTE – those with highest risk (e.g. in patients about to undergo orthopaedic surgery) require rapid induction.

7.5 What is the general method for changing a patient's warfarin dose to ensure their INR is in range?

Simply to recommend to the patient that they increase/decrease their daily dose (up-titration/ down-titration)

7.6 What is the approximate average daily dose of warfarin taken by low-risk patients?

Perhaps 4 or 5mg on alternate days

7.7 What is the approximate average daily dose of warfarin taken by high-risk patients?

Maybe 6mg a day

7.8 What patient factors influence the dose of warfarin?

Age, use of alcohol, heart and renal disease, weight gain, diarrhoea and vomiting (Table 7.4)

8.1 Why are NOACs preferred to traditional agents in certain indications?

They are at least as effective (sometimes more) and safer (causing fewer bleeds).

8.2 What medical factors must be considered in the use of NOACs?

The practitioner needs to be aware of (at least!) renal function and co-medications, as these may be cautions and/or contra-indications.

8.3 What is the difference between a NICE clinical guideline and a technology appraisal?

A clinical guideline makes recommendations regarding particular indications such as after orthopaedic surgery and AF. A technology appraisal makes recommendations about the use of specific drugs.

8.4 Which of the NOACs can be used to prevent VTEs after orthopaedic surgery?
NICE has licensed dabigatran, rivaroxaban and apixaban for this indication. In the future, other NOACs may become licensed.

8.5 People with AF are not at a very high risk of VTE, so why do they need to be anticoagulated?
AF is a major cause of stroke.

9.1 What is the antidote for excess heparin?
Protamine sulphate

9.2 What are the first actions in cases of excess warfarin or a NOAC?
For warfarin, stop taking the drug, obtain an INR, and give vitamin K. For a NOAC, just stop the drug. Other actions will follow (depending on haemorrhage).

9.3 What are the treatments for life-threatening haemorrhage?
Blood transfusion and blood components such as prothrombin complex concentrate

9.4 Which commonly prescribed drugs interact with warfarin?
Antibiotics, cytotoxic chemotherapy, statins, amiodarone

Answers to case studies

Case Study 1

The major laboratory abnormality is the high level of D-dimers, which may be caused by numerous factors, such as atherosclerosis and cancer. However, the woman has diabetes, and so this may be the cause. But the key clinical question is whether or not the woman has a DVT, and if so, this may be the reason for the raised D-dimers. Certainly, she is obese, is over 60, and has several clinical indicators of DVT. So, in the absence of the gold standard tool, ultrasonography, the only question is whether or not to give a LMWH. On balance, many practitioners would, but would also ensure an ultrasound be performed as soon as possible to help confirm/exclude a DVT.

Case Study 2

This woman's treatment is standard, but the nosebleeds are worrying. Investigation of this reveals thrombocytopenia (platelet count <100) but a normal APTT ratio. Therefore it looks like the problem is heparin-induced thrombocytopenia. Treatment of this is to remove the heparin, and start her on any of the three NOACs. Indeed, if she had been placed on a NOAC in the first place, this case would not have presented.

Case Study 3

This woman is at moderately high risk of an additional VTE because of her history, a present risk (pregnancy), and the presence of FVL. The anti-Factor Xa result is at the bottom end of therapeutic range (i.e. as if she actually has a VTE) but is low for a prophylactic dose (i.e. in VTE prevention). The test should be repeated, and if confirmed the dose (20mg of the LMWH daily) should probably be maintained as she is at a more than average risk of a repeat VTE.

Case Study 4

The elderly woman's target INR is 3.5, so her first three results are acceptable. The fourth (INR 4.1) is only just outside the target range of 3–4, and the dosing officer is rewarded for keeping the dose stable as the INR comes back in range on 3rd September. However, the result that follows is unacceptable, and following the previous high level of 4.1, demands a reduction of the dose to 3mg daily but 4mg on Wednesday and Sunday (i.e. 3.25mg daily over the week).

Case Study 5

The CHA_2DS_2VASc, HAS-BLED and $SAMe-TT_2R_2$ scores apply, as described in Figure 8.2 and Table 8.6. This man's CHA_2DS_2VASc score is 4 (hypertension, age over 75, and other vascular disease), and his HAS-BLED score is 2 (hypertension and elderly), although use of aspirin brings this to 3. However, as his CHA_2DS_2VASc score exceeds his HAS-BLED score, he would need to be on OAC, and so the aspirin would be stopped. His $SAMe-TT_2R_2$ score is 3 (Me = the chronic medical diseases of peripheral vascular disease and prostate disease, and R = non-Caucasian), and so he should be on a NOAC. Incidentally, being obese and elderly, in addition to having peripheral vascular disease, and so likely to have mobility problems, a NOAC may also be preferred on social grounds, as a VKA would need to be monitored with an INR. This would therefore require him to travel, or the anticoagulant service to visit him at home. Any of the three NOACs would be applicable, but before doing so, an assessment of renal function would be called for. Incidentally, his blood pressure is above target (140/90) so this should be addressed, perhaps by increasing the amlodipine, or by adding a second drug, such as an ACEI/ARB or a diuretic. But beforehand, renal function is again an issue.

Case Study 6

This profile is very concerning as the INR is all over the place with no clear pattern. There is one dangerously high INR leading to fears of possibly important haemorrhage. The ability of this patient to understand instructions to self-dose must be questioned. The duration of anticoagulation is short, implying a transient risk factor, and so it may be safer to take the patient off warfarin and replace it with a NOAC. The reason for OAC is unclear, but only rivaroxaban is licensed for the treatment of VTE (the others are licensed only for prevention).

Case Study 7

The patient (clearly on warfarin) seems to have induced his own surface haemorrhage and would probably be worried that he may have additional bleeds, may lose his sight, or even the eye. Nevertheless, it is reassuring that his INR is entirely normal and this is important as it will provide some reassurance (to both of you). Some may be tempted to reduce his dose of warfarin to reduce the risk of more bleeding; this is quite possibly what the patient has in mind. However, this will inevitably increase his risk of thrombosis, and if this precipitates a DVT, PE or thrombotic stroke, it could be hard to defend.

Case Study 8

The high INR is clearly actionable according to Table 9.2, i.e. stop warfarin. Consider vitamin K oral 1.0mg; re-test next day. However, with the history of haematuria certainly give vitamin K, and re-test daily until the INR approaches 4 or 5, and then resume warfarin. Also consider reducing the dose for a day or two. But the patient must be probed for possible causes. If the loss of blood seems considerable, then take a full blood count and act on the results, e.g. consider blood transfusion. It therefore follows that, in the case of the latter, secondary care will be involved. Don't forget to look for thrombocytopenia (platelet count <100), and the possibility of drug interactions. Depending on the reason for being on an OAC your consultation will also provide the opportunity to discuss the pros and cons of one of the NOACs.

Case Study 9

It seems likely that the haemorrhage is due to the rivaroxaban, so that in the absence of a precipitating event (such as a co-medication), options are returning to warfarin, or a different NOAC. Of the two, apixaban has a better haemorrhagic profile than dabigatran. In clinical trials, dabigatran was associated with 20% fewer major bleeds, whilst apixaban was linked to 31% fewer bleeds, although this difference is not statistically significant. A likely dose is 2.5mg twice a day.

Glossary

Acenocoumarol: a vitamin K antagonist, sometimes used in place of warfarin

Activated partial thromboplastin time (APTT): the time taken for plasma to clot that relies on the presence of various coagulation factors including Factors VIII and X

Activated partial thromboplastin time ratio (APTT ratio): the ratio between the APTT whilst the patient is on heparin compared to the APTT when not on heparin

Antiphospholipid antibodies: an autoimmune and thrombophilic condition where the patient is at increased risk of VTE

Anti-thrombin: a major inhibitor of the coagulation pathway

Apixaban: a non-vitamin K antagonist oral anticoagulant and possible replacement for warfarin and/or heparin in certain circumstances

Aspirin: the most commonly used anti-platelet drug

British National Formulary (BNF): The major pharmaceutical textbook giving information and recommendations about all drugs used in the NHS

Coagulation: the process of clot formation

Clopidogrel: an anti-platelet drug and so alternative to aspirin

Cytotoxic drug: any drug that has a toxic effect on cells

Dabigatran: a non-vitamin K antagonist oral anticoagulant and possible replacement for warfarin and/or heparin in certain circumstances

D-dimers: the products of a clot digested by plasmin in the process of fibrinolysis

Deep vein thrombosis (DVT): a clot in a vein in the leg

Direct thrombin inhibitor: an anticoagulant whose mode of action is to act directly on thrombin, and so inhibit its action.

DOAC: a direct-acting oral coagulant

Edoxaban: a non-vitamin K antagonist oral anticoagulant and possible replacement for warfarin and/or heparin in certain circumstances

Embolectomy: surgical removal of a clot

Embolus: a clot or fragment of a clot (plural – emboli)

Epidemiology: the study of disease in populations (as opposed to the individual)

Factor V: a coagulation factor important in the initiation of coagulation. It is the object of inhibition by protein C

Factor V Leiden: a mutant form of Factor V that resists inhibition by protein C and so promotes thrombosis. It is the most common cause of thrombophilia

Factor VII: a coagulation protein often used to treat haemorrhage

Factor VIII: the coagulation factor lacking in haemophilia

Factor X: a coagulation factor that is inhibited by anti-thrombin and LMWH. Activated Factor Xa can be used to assess the impact of LMWH

Factor Xa inhibitors: an anticoagulant whose mode of action is to act directly on coagulation Factor Xa, and so inhibit its action.

Fibrin: a blood protein, derived from fibrinogen, that forms a mesh to trap platelets and so form a clot

Fibrinogen: a major coagulation protein, synthesised by the liver, that is converted by thrombin into fibrin

Fibrinolysis: the dissolution of fibrin, i.e. clot removal

Fondaparinux: a very precisely targeted drug that mimics the action of LMWH but is far more sensitive, specific and reliable

Graduated elastic compression stockings (GECS): a non-drug therapy that aims to reduce the risk of thrombosis or its recurrence

Haemophilia: a haemorrhagic disorder the results from a lack of coagulation Factor VIII

Haemoptysis: the coughing up of blood

Haemorrhage: inappropriate bleeding

Haemostasis: the balance between the forces of coagulation (forming a clot) and the forces inhibiting that process and also removing the clot (fibrinolysis)

Heparin: an anticoagulant that must be given through the skin

Heparin-induced thrombocytopenia (HIT): a low platelet count that is caused by heparin

Heterozygous: describing a pair of genes, in which one is dominant and one is recessive

International Normalised Ratio (INR): the ratio between the time blood or plasma takes to clot whilst the patient is taking warfarin and the time taken to clot whilst not on warfarin

Lyse: to cause destruction of cells by lysins

Low molecular weight heparin (LMWH): a safer, more recently developed version of heparin

National Institute for Health and Care Excellence (NICE): a government body that issues recommendations regarding the use of drugs, such as in the prevention and treatment of VTE in surgery

National Patient Safety Agency (NPSA): a government body that issues actions and instructions regarding Trust management of anticoagulation

NOAC: non-vitamin K antagonist oral anticoagulant

Oestrogen: steroid hormones that promote the female characteristics of the body

Parenteral: a route of drug delivery through the skin (i.e., an injection)

Phenidione: a vitamin K antagonist, sometimes used in place of warfarin

Plasmin: the enzyme that digests fibrin in the process of fibrinolysis

Platelet: a tiny blood cell that forms a clot (thrombus) when aggregated with fibrin

Post-thrombotic syndrome: the long-term consequences of DVT, manifesting as venous ulceration, varicose veins, dermatitis, etc.

Prophylaxis: prevention

Protein C: a major inhibitor of the coagulation pathway

Protein S: a major inhibitor of the coagulation pathway

Prothrombin (PT): a major coagulation protein, synthesised by the liver, that gives rise to thrombin

Prothrombinase: a complex of Factor Xa and other components that together make a 'super-enzyme' that converts prothrombin to thrombin

Prothrombin time: a laboratory measure of the time plasma takes to form a clot that is dependent on prothrombin but also some other coagulation factors (e.g. Factor V)

Pulmonary embolus: clot in a vessel of the lung

Rivaroxaban: a non-vitamin K antagonist oral anticoagulant and possible replacement for warfarin and/or heparin in certain circumstances

Thrombin: the blood enzyme that converts fibrinogen to fibrin

Thrombocytopenia: generally held to be a platelet count less than 100

Thrombolysis: the process of clot dissolution

Thrombophilia: a condition where there is an increased tendency to form clots

Thrombosis committee: a body of Trust staff who take responsibility for all matters regarding prophylaxis and treatment of VTE

Thrombus: clot

Tissue plasminogen activator (tPA): the protein that is needed to generate plasmin

Unfractionated heparin (UFH): 'old style' heparin, as opposed to the newer LMWH

Venous thromboembolism (VTE): a clot in a vein

Vitamin K antagonist (VKA): a group of drugs whose anticoagulant effect is due to their antagonism of the metabolism of vitamin K requiring molecules

Warfarin: a VKA anticoagulant that may be taken orally

Index